Broken Trails
Ambushed By Cancer
3rd Ed.

Sara M. Slayton and Paul D. Heckman

For Each Other

I believe...
...that imagination is stronger
than knowledge,
...that myth is more potent
than history,
...that dreams are more powerful
than facts,
...that hope always triumphs
over experience,
...that laughter is the only cure
for grief,
...that love is stronger
than death.

The Storyteller's Creed
Robert Fulghum

Permanent Cowgirl

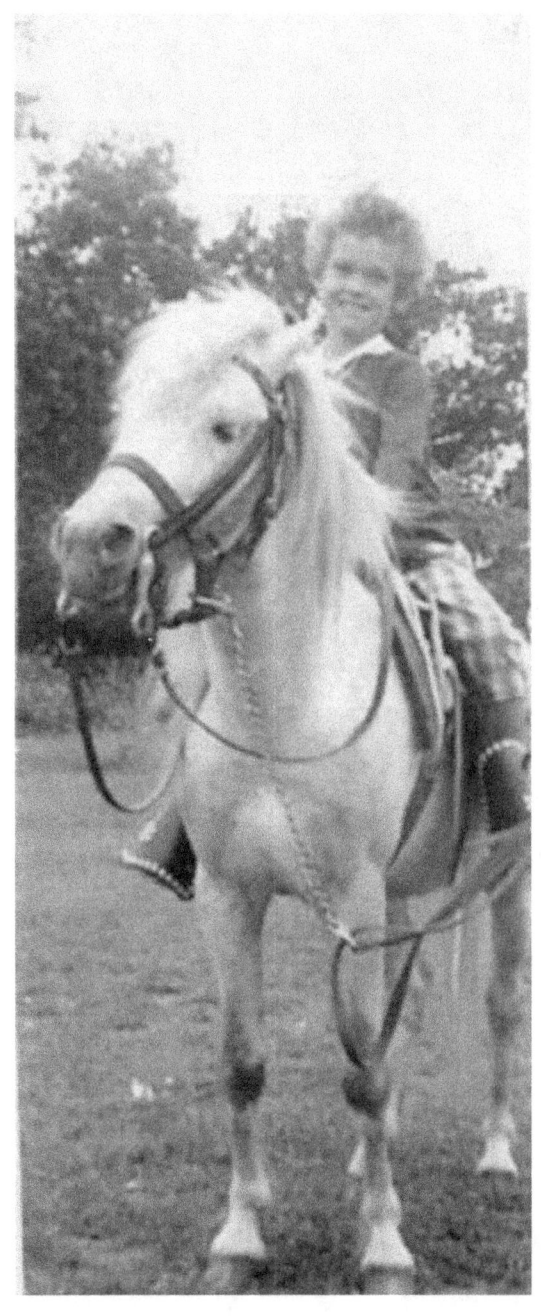

Table of Contents

Trail's End 1
Little Girl 3
The One To Have 6
Ear To The Glass 9
Fleisch 12
My Misfortune Is Not Your Warning 14
Math 15
Boomer's Got A Question 17
The Beast 19
Tropical Cancer 23
Bosom Buddies 24
Bargaining 27
Quotes 29
Flora's Tale 31
Is It Time? 37
I'm Guessing 39
Cancer Logic 40
Ms. Trauma 43
Faced With The Prospect 46
Tides 54
Dr. De-i-ety 57
Distractions And The Disconnect 59
Coverage 62
Mea Culpa 64

The Play: Until We Meet Again 65

TRAIL'S END

Sara Slayton

When I was a little girl my friends and I would often put on a "show". We would gather together the usual bunch of reluctant volunteers: younger siblings, moms, pets, as our captive audience. Often, we had the bravado to charge admission to these little bits of amusement, maybe a penny or a piece of candy. In elaborate pieces of costume, we would share our dubious talents until the dogs wandered off with the toddlers shortly behind them. Eventually, the faithful mothers, who had to get back to the serious business of the day, would clap politely. This was our signal to wind things up.

We staged many of these neighborhood productions in a summer's time. We danced in oversized high heels; we did magic tricks with props purchased from the Woolworth's store; we sang silly songs in plucky, if not tuneful voices, and we often dressed up our pets – accepting the applause for their tricks.

We imagined ourselves to be legends in our own time and dreamed of illustrious futures. In those days we yearned for the ability to see who we would become and to know what adventures awaited us. In our minds we became famous, but humble, champions. We were certain that our future lives would be full of chivalrous and daring deeds.

No one among us imagined the likelihood of illness, nor did we have a frame of reference in which to place such a concept. We knew someday we would grow old and die but that was a vaporous notion at best.

My greatest hope and ambition as a child was to become a cowgirl. It was the age of television westerns and I was charmed by every detail of the genre. I liked the clothes, I loved the horses, and the appeal of a maverick attitude was potent for a little independent girl. I was sure I would become the kindly rancher's steely-eyed daughter, who would rescue animals and eat beans from a tin plate. Not only did I believe this was possible, I had faith that it would come true.

I took this vision with me everywhere and when it was my turn to take the stage I did so as the rancher's daughter. I stood behind the blanket we hung across the garage door in my tooled, leather-look boots while wearing a fringed vest I had made from a brown grocery bag. I sauntered out to center stage and crooned my favorite anthem, 'Home on the Range' often adding a few whoops and hollers to underscore my character.

Never once did I imagine the trail's end.

LITTLE GIRL

Sara Slayton

I sit, curled into an upright fetal position. My heels tuck up against my butt and my chin rests on my knees. I am reminded of those coral flamingos at the zoo. They stand at the edge of a pool in a controlled rain forest. They are always there but I've never actually witnessed one move.

I can hold myself in my own arms. It occurs to me that I don't take up much space these days. Across the room I see my childhood rocking chair. Made of pine slats and nearly 50 years old, it has most recently been used by my grandson. At seven, he is now a bit big for the chair...if not in stature, surely in his perception of his own maturity. I wonder about my own perceptions. Would I fit in that chair?

One's body image is a curious thing. I used to know instinctively how much space I needed to move around, how much room I needed on a bench for instance, or what size clothes to try on. Now, I am confused. I try to judge these things and I'm not accurate. It's when I misjudge – when my jeans fall down around my hips, that I get a sense of my changed significance in the physical world. If I take up less space, if I put less of a burden on the earth does that make some kind of difference?

When I was a child, my father nicknamed me the "Mighty Mite". He said it was because I was tough and stubborn and had a low center of gravity. He liked to think I couldn't be pushed over easily. When I look back on the photos of my childhood I can see he was right. I weighed over nine pounds at birth and was two weeks overdue. I practically sprang from my mother's womb, in a record short labor, with a healthy scream and a head full of fine, dark hair.

It was a robust start. I did everything early – walked, talked, ate solid food. By the time I was two years old I had rolls of baby fat that made little sweaty folds at my elbows and my knees. I ate anything set before me and I loved corn on the cob. My hair was thick, my eyes were clear and I was always tan. I remember liking my sturdy legs and priding myself on being able to carry heavy things.

I was so comfortable in my skin. I knew the heat of it when I ran, the taste of it on a hot afternoon, the sweet smell of my own hair when it fell over my face.

....

My first course of chemo was a nightmare. I continued working and scheduled my treatments for Thursday afternoons. I didn't teach on Friday so I was able to take three days to cope with the worst of the treatment after-math. I found that when my body was poisoned by the chemicals it reacted by rejecting the pestilence with a no-nonsense approach. Every system in my body began to slap down the invaders. My nose ran, my eyes watered, my bowels emptied, and I spent the first day and a half after treatment vomiting. I learned to prepare for the onslaught by eating as much as I could for the 24 hours preceding treatment. Anything that looked good to me on Wednesday was fair game. Of course that plan eventually failed as my appetite dried up.

One day, with three or four treatments under my belt, and having braved the latest battle with the "side effects", I crept into my bed. I slept for the next 16 hours. I woke in a warm, still room. I could hear the oscillating fan and its path would pass over me every 20 seconds. It was a gentle routine. The breeze was scented by the room around me, and something else. I have always had a keen sense of smell. What I detected now was some sort of automotive. The heavy musk of lead, of something tainted. This was not good. This was the smell of danger. I opened my eyes to realize that what I was smelling was my own arm. I was cradling my head and the smell of chemo poison was oozing out of my skin in nearly invisible, deadly dew.

....

Some days now, when I've been working in the garden, my skin gets moist. I put my arm up to my face and take a deep breath. I lick the inside of my elbow. I smell warm and I taste sweet again, like roasted corn with real butter.

THE ONE TO HAVE
Paul Dominic Heckman

(Since our first publication in 2007 I, too, have had a bout with cancer. Less dangerous than Sara's, but no more deserved.)

"If you have to have cancer, this is the one to have." I heard it dozens of times – doctors, nurses, oncologists, radiation technicians, visitors – it was meant to be reassuring. It wasn't. Not then.

"If you have to have cancer…"

That's where I got stuck. This development arose how exactly? Thyroid cancer. You know, the one to have if you have to have cancer. Of course the explanation is that the incidence of thyroid cancer has become much more frequent, and the treatment is statistically quite successful. So. Aren't you happy?

No. I'm still on the "have to have" part. Did Sara "have to have" cancer? Why? Why were hers, statistically, really not the ones to have? Who or what determines this bestowal?

I'd had a sore neck and had gone for an MRI. A couple days later, "No, your bones are just getting older. We did, however, notice a suspicious darkness in your thyroid area." (I hear things differently from others: If the darkness was suspicious, it had every reason to be; it had no business being there). We would investigate. Biopsy. That was a word that had never appeared on my schedule before. I was not worried or scared or even terribly affected. Sara had paved this road through cancer, and hers wasn't even the one to have! I truly was not afraid. We were calm, but firm in our reaction. Breathe. Deeply. Slowly.

However, after a few days I did need and began to find some assurance from various sources. Sara, of course, was what I needed. And her family, too, once again mustered to shoulder this weight. But it also played in my head that "this was the one to have...", and I became somewhat pleased at the thought. Well, I had to have some kind of cancer, I guess, so why not the best one? The idea of best is implied by the phrase "one to have". Actually, of course, no cancer is the one to have. And that "have to have" idea kept gnawing at me. Until I realized that the phrase is faulty. No one has to have cancer. Sometimes we just do. Certainly there are many valid and unavoidable reasons that cancer stirs and awakens. But it is not necessary to anything but itself. "Growth for growth's sake is the ideology of the cancer cell." (Edward Abbey)

After Sara's first bout we, of course, looked into what defines this terrifying concept. One of the things I had learned about the disease is that cancer cells are always present in each of us. It lives benignly in our bodies all the time. It's always there. But something triggers it to grow.

I could not think of a single reason why someone would have to have cancer. In fact, no one HAS to have cancer. It appears for many reasons and we must continue to look for causes and solutions, but the epiphany is that a positive, proactive approach to cancer's appearance helps. And the advancements in prevention, treatments, and therapy options have continued steadily so that, now, our 1988 experience seems primitive. I learned about cancer and lived through it twice, now three times, with a wonderful person who did not have to have cancer. She just did. I just did. It is our approach to it – OK, well, let's do what's next – that made the fight more bearable. What more can one do than the best one can do? So we write, we educate, we donate time and money, we support and encourage, we comfort and reassure. Each of us suffers and fears life's turns to varying degrees at various times, for short and long periods and sometimes for life. But our love for each other and those around us is reason enough for Sara and me to respond with a calmness and strength that comes from letting go. The idea is as simple and as complex as it sounds. We need to examine our culture and evaluate our rituals. We need to reduce preconceptions of cancer's history and our fears of powerlessness. This requires truly not fearing the past or dreading the future, but doing what we can for ourselves and others to be safe and secure, acting calmly and positively, handling the moments. Breathe deeply. Slowly, and let go.

It is an unusual approach for many of us. But it helps and doesn't hurt. When we hear a diagnosis we form an immediate reaction, a general response, and a long-term attitude. I contend that if you have to have an attitude, this is the one to have.

EAR TO THE GLASS

Sara Slayton

When I was three years old we got our first television. It was
a bulky piece of furniture with a very small screen. We got
three channels and they played for limited hours each day.
Often I would turn on the TV and find what was called a 'test
pattern'. I recall that it looked like a target and played a
single, relentless tone. At the end of each day's programming
the national anthem would play across a screen of the
billowing flag...then a pause and the return of the test
pattern. We would turn off the set and the picture would
fade into a disappearing white dot. It was all very simple and
predictable.

I was the first generation raised on television. I got my hair
set in pin curls every Saturday night while we watched
Bonanza. I would come running from outside when I heard
Captain Bob ask, "What time is it kids?" I was a faithful
viewer of Captain Kangaroo and thought that I might like to
marry Dancing Bear some day.

I also enjoyed the countless half hour sitcoms. I could whistle
along at the beginning of the Andy Griffith show. I could
name all the characters on Wagon Train, and I laughed at the
antics of Lucy and Ricky, Ethel and Fred.

I recall one episode of the 'I Love Lucy' show in which Lucy
suspected that Ricky was having an affair with another
woman in the apartment building. There was no truth to this
of course, but Lucy and Ethel were determined to listen in on
the conversation between Ricky and the "other woman".
They went into the basement and opened up the furnace
vents, allowing them to listen in on every apartment in the
building. It seems that I learned several ways of trying to
listen in on other's conversations from television. The most
popular method of course was to put a drinking glass against

the wall and put your ear up to it. I attempted this several times when I was trying to spy on my older sister in the next room of my house. But whatever glass I tried it seemed I could only hear a rushing noise, similar to when you put a seashell to your ear. Then the sound would be drowned out by my own heartbeat.

I awake and it is twilight. It seems as if it is always twilight these days. There is a very soft play of last light on the curtains. I lie still, watching it creep across the dirty carpet. How long have I slept this time? Sometimes I confuse dawn with dusk. But now I hear voices. It is my husband playing with our grandson in the other room. Their play is robust, but I can tell they are 'keeping it down' because grandma needs her rest. Silly voices, giggly voices, voices that make me smile, absorbed in their play. They are fighting a battle. Winning and losing, but always coming out as heroes. Always ready to face another day, another battle...renewed and hopeful and ready for whatever comes next.

I do not stir. I do not disturb the energy in this house. Is this the way it will be when I'm gone? If I die from this crazy illness will these voices continue? I lie there playing some sort of macabre version of "if a tree falls in the woods and no one is there to hear it..."

There is a way that human beings can become invisible. I have discovered that now. It has to do with lying very still and simply listening. It is a strange way of eavesdropping on your own life. I can actually wander through my own house in my mind, unseen and not disturbing so much as a mote of dust. I can look it over, pretty much without passion or even a very strong connection. Somehow I can become detached. That's when I disappear.

II start to speak about this phenomenon to my counselor,

but as I do the rushing sound comes to my ears and my heart starts to beat too hard. The experience becomes a hot memory that rushes up in my throat. There is a painful and audible catch in my voice, my breath. This always leads to tears. They sting my eyes and run down my face. I watch as they fall with a soft thud onto the vinyl couch. It occurs to me that I am leaving my DNA there. It becomes a target-shaped puddle that I view with detachment as a single relentless tone begins to sound in my brain. I switch it off... the connection to life, the pain, and the laugh track all fade into a disappearing white dot.

FLEISCH
Sara Slayton

When I was a child I spent a lot of time with my maternal grandparents. From them I learned about being German. They were stout people, solid people, and they liked a hearty meal. We drank whole milk in those days and often used heavy cream on things such as bowls full of raspberries from the garden. We liberally sprinkled white sugar on everything from fried doughnuts to stalks of rhubarb. We fried foods in butter and we used lard to make our pie crusts. Slabs of cheese were served with every meal, including breakfast when the cheese was often melted over a piece of warm apple pie. The anchor of any meal in that household was the meat – wurst, or fleisch as it was called.

For many years when I was growing up, my father worked for Oscar Mayer and Company. It was factory work, mean and hard, but one of the benefits was being able to shop at the Employee's Market. I remember this as a barren little storefront attached to the main plant. It smelled of wieners. Men in long white aprons waited on my mother. We would walk in front of the refrigerated cases, peering over rows, mounds, and tubes of pink flesh. My mother would make her careful choices, thankful for the discount we received for my father's labors. Sometimes we would purchase 'mistakes'...wieners that were longer than buns, or big bologna that was sliced too thick for the cellophane packages. These purchases were always unplanned, and, therefore somewhat exciting, and they were the best deals in our monthly meat budget. Processed cold meat was a staple of my daily diet and I loved all things pork and beef.

When I was ten years old my grandfather suffered a fatal stroke. It was not until many years later that I realized his habit of eating lard and wurst sandwiches might have contributed to his early death. I was half grown before anyone started talking about things like nitrites, or preservatives, salt content, or animal fat.

When I was diagnosed with cancer I fell prey to the haunting questions of most patients. I searched for the things that had brought me to the edge of this particular darkness. I tried to pin down the culprit, the moment, the poor decision. They say we are what we eat. Did I ingest cancer? Was it one patty too many? One fatal slab of too-thick sliced bacon?

Sometimes I imagine that the color of my cancer is a pale bologna and the aftertaste of chemo is akin to charred wieners.

MY MISFORTUNE IS NOT YOUR WARNING
Paul Dominic Heckman

"It's a sign from God telling us all to slow down."
"God has a special purpose for us."
"God never gives us more than we can handle."
"It's God's way of telling us, 'Trust Me!'"

I heard a lot about what God wants when I was diagnosed with thyroid cancer in 2006. My favorite is, "Boy, this sure is a wake-up call from God!" How so? For whom? Who are all these narcoleptics who keep needing a rude interruption from their slumber? I don't mean to be cynical, but really, *what you get from my diagnosis* is a wake-up call? Glad I could help. Look, I don't mean to be ungrateful but sometimes a cancer is just a cancer. That's always a possibility. It isn't some heavenly message. If, in fact, it were God's way of sending messages, wouldn't it be a good idea for us to learn the lesson once and for all and stay alert so innocent people wouldn't have to be the envelope for God's behavior memos? Attributing serious danger and a simple hotel service to God's preferred methods is insulting to everyone involved. This goes for natural disasters and wide-spread diseases as well. So here's my advice. Behave because it's in everyone's best interest, and spend your time, money, and energy looking for solutions to our worldly problems. That will make God happy.

MATH

Sara Slayton

I vaguely remember hearing one of the doctors ask, "Do you really want to hear this?" "Sure," I replied. What could he possibly have to tell me that I hadn't already tried to ignore? Whenever one of these guys explained something, I was immediately transported back to my under-graduate math class.

I don't know if there is a good time of day to learn math when you are single, 19 years old, and more than a bit distracted, but certainly any time before noon was pushing it for me. When one combined an 8:00 a.m. math class with the expectation of daily attendance, a real issue was at hand. I was preparing to be an elementary school teacher. There was one required math course that all teacher candidates had to pass. The odds seemed to be in my favor, but the content was more than contrary for me. I took the class three times before I mastered that passing grade. Twice I withdrew at about mid-semester, when the language of the content went beyond what I could possibly comprehend. When I finally passed the course it was because I had memorized the first eight weeks of material. Succeeding in that class didn't leave me with a sense of pride or mastery, only a sense that I had cleared some sort of hurdle. I was lazy, and disinclined, and easily felt comfortable with the idea that I would never use this stuff in my real life.
When I catch up with the doctor, he is speaking the language of my math professor: "There is an 80% chance that this thing is malignant." "The surgery is successful about 70% of the time." "Only 2 out of 5 patients survive this type of cancer after the first 5 years." Now he's got my attention. This is a language I think I understand, and that scares me at several levels.

A year has passed since that conversation. The 'thing' was malignant and I survived the surgery. So much for that part of the word problem known as my life. I guess it means that I was fortunate to be in the majority, or is it the minority? Now that 2 out of 5 piece is starting to puzzle me, to plague me. Since a whole year has passed I don't quite know where we are in this problem. I keep picturing a group of 5, skinny, hairless figures on a graph. Has one of them disappeared? Is it only one? What does that mean for the remaining 4 of us? Are my odds better or worse today?

Maybe I should have paid more attention back in that math class, it seems as if the figures are now desperately relevant. But somehow, a piece of me embraces the bliss of ignorance. At times one can know too much.

BOOMER'S GOT A QUESTION

Paul Dominic Heckman

Momma said it's dangerous; daddy said it too,
But the doctors and nurses assure me the purpose
Is only to help pull me through.
If I ask if it's safe now
Well, they smile and they wink, as if to say,
"In this place, man,
It's better not to think."

I'm just worried and wonderin' how bad can turn
out good?
Does radiation somehow know
To do the things we say we know it should
With its luminescent glow?

Momma says it's painless; daddy nods his head,
And the doctors and nurses assure me the curse is
Being sick means at least I'm not dead.
When I ask them what has changed,
Why is nuking me O.K.?
I see their faces look ashamed
Before they look away.

I'm just worried and wonderin' how you came to decide;
Does radiation really find
The senseless, scary growth I have inside?
How can evil be so kind?

I'm just worried and wonderin' about what I used to hear;
Can radiation be all right?
Can something we all once claimed to fear
Be cast in such a light?

So here I am just asking, not to contradict,
Can the doctors and nurses assure me the worst is
The best they can do for the sick?
Yes, I still have some questions
As they place the shield of lead;
Can something bring me back to life
That's meant to make us dead?

I'm just worried and wonderin' about what I used to hear;
Can radiation be all right?
Can something we all once claimed to fear
Be cast in such a light?

From the musical play Until We Meet Again
By Sara M. Slayton and Paul D. Heckman

THE BEAST
Sara Slayton

The beast has returned. A man-child told me of its approach.
He had not seen it before, so it frightened him. He told me
that he saw it coming up from behind me, behind the curve of
my back and he believed it was after my soft, belly flesh. The
last time it had come head on, going for my throat. This was a
newer and more subtle approach. Don't get me wrong, I did
have some hints of its reappearance. A sort of gnawing had
been awake in my belly for a month, but I wanted to believe it
was something else – anything else – but I knew.

The man-child told me that the only way to rid myself of the
beast was to grow intimate with it, to know every detail of its
makeup. He also told me that he couldn't help me with that. I
would have to rely on older and wiser advisors than he. So I
drove across the prairie searching out people who knew my
monster, its idiosyncrasies, and its fears. They were men who
handled other people's beasts on a daily basis. They were not
afraid of them because they were not their own. These
detached sages touched my body and they gave me counsel
and then I was armed with their knowledge. The proposed
battle plan was a three-pronged type of aggression – first by
knife, then by poison, then by fire. All three phases of the
attack would rob me of strength and endurance and in the end,
it was impossible to tell who would come out alive, the beast
or me.

Since then the days have been wintery. This weather better
suits the beast than it does me. The chill reaches deep
inside me. I have no blankets that can keep it out.

The beast corners me in stillness, causing a sense of panic that rises in my throat to choke off my breathing with its bile-like taste. My first reaction is to freeze, not fight. But the monster is clever. It does not strike right away. It snarls in the corner, keeping me trapped and making me picture my own defeat.

Damn this animal that grows in the heart of me! It not only stalks me but it sniffs around everyone I love. Only two years ago a similar beast took the life of my father. It bites and tears and takes down friends – actors, mothers, teachers – leaving them bald and maimed and scarred. It leaves them for dead. But some of them rise again, growing stubble in place of hair, and wearing pink ribbons that reflect the scars on their bodies. Some rise and some fall, what does that mean for me?

The hot breath of the beast pulses in my ear at night, making me restless even though I am weary beyond reason. I am becoming nocturnal, somehow fearing the night because it belongs to darker beings. And then it lulls me to sleep during the day, keeping me from being active, and strong, and productive. Its methods of attack are cunning and diverse.

It is afraid of some people. It fears my husband, slinking away whenever it sees him approach. It fears his strength and the strength I take from him. But it is even getting braver around him. It has begun to nip at his heels and to cause him moments of grief and self-doubt. In the end, my husband and I know who the beast is after, and we know that ultimately I will be the one to have to face it.

I'm making myself toxic in order to become poisonous to the creature. I pump the poison into my body one drip at a time, opening a vein in defense. The beast sniffs around me, but sometimes now it no longer finds a human scent.

Each day I go to my arena to fight the beast. There are many others there with their own creatures to defeat. Many of the other warriors are older than I. They often appear weaker than I, yet they rise to fight when their names are called. They go into the dark room and don their lead shields against the fire that can kill – either the beasts or them. There are numbers of people who have fought the brothers of my beast. Most of them don't hold out for more than a five year battle. I wonder how good a warrior I really am.

I disrobe, lie down, put my hands over my head and visualize the creature's demise. I see myself as an old woman dancing on the Cliffs of Mohr. Sensing a future seems to stave off, or at least slow down the beast's approach.

My body is smaller than when I started the fight. It is not that I have grown lean with strength from the battle, but that parts of me are missing – birth parts, trust parts, cavalier parts, innocent parts. How can such a small body fight such grueling battles? It's as if all the air has been let out of me and my muscles and strength lie dormant under a progressively drying and thinning layer of skin. I dream of speed and movement that I can no longer achieve. I imagine myself running, or dancing, or bouncing a baby. I cannot work while I am being hunted. I must be vigilant.

The fight is very expensive. It takes so much money, so much effort, so much pain, so much trust, so much patience. The costs of survival are dear.

People know that I am in the battle. They see it on my face – a look of the victim, which is bewildering to the strong. They see it in my diminished body. They notice the poisonous armor that I must wear at all times. They are not quite sure what to do for me. They encourage, or they commiserate, or they get angry and withdraw.

Between battles I try to fortify myself. I eat, I sleep, hoping that these simple restorative measures will somehow make a difference in the next day's battle.

Sometimes I come to consciousness from a deep, unnatural sleep to hear the voices of my home. I hear a song, a laugh, the soft breaths of sleep. But I hear them now as if I am no longer a part of them, only an eavesdropper. I wonder what this home would be without me. If it could be without me?

Then there are the moments of delusion, of denial, when I can nearly ignore its presence. I go about my business as if the beast had never come into my life. Then a gentle whirring sets off a deep stabbing pain in my belly flesh – its target.

I close my eyes, waiting for enough weariness to shut down my senses, my thoughts, my fears. A blessed weariness without the beastly nightmare battles.

TROPICAL CANCER

Paul Dominic Heckman

[Chorus intro]
On Col O Gee, On Col O Gee,
They look for signs inside of me.
On Col O Gee, On Col O Gee,
Oh what size fruit's inside of me?

Bio Op See, Bio Op See,
Oh what size fruit's inside of me?
Bio Op See, Bio Op See,
They look for signs inside of me.

They are so wise, to name the size —
A lemon, a lime, a grape this time?
They are astute, their point is moot —
Wow! You've got a ripe grapefruit!

An orange, a cherry, a huckleberry,
What's on the tree inside of me?
A mango, pineapple, I sound like Snapple,
Oh ya it's Strawberry Kiwi.

On Col O Gee, Bio Op See,
A citrus fruit menagerie.
Bio Op See, On Col O Gee,
This fruit is not so good for me.

Bio Op See, On Col O Gee,
This fruit is not so good for me.
On Col O Gee, Bio Op See,
Harvest this mess inside of me.

From the musical play Until We Meet Again
By Sara M. Slayton and Paul D. Heckman

BOSOM BUDDIES
Sara Slayton

My sister Linda is one of the most gentle souls I have known. She feels the breath of life somehow more keenly than most of us. If often chafes her because it comes too strongly, too roughly. When she was born she started crying and she didn't stop for six months. She was what was called 'colicky' by the neighborhood women. I think she just knew it was a harsh world before the rest of us.

When she first came into contact with the brutal world of public education she was blind-sided by it. She had no context in which to put much of the behavior she witnessed. She walked gently into a lion's den. There she found Rosine, who turned out to be the nemesis of her early childhood. In a day when little girls were named Janice and Debbie, Rosine seemed as exotic as her name. There was a worldliness about her that she wore like a cloak of superiority, even in first grade. She was bright, quick, articulate, and mean spirited. My sister looked like a victim to Rosine. She once told my sister that she admired her new coat. I remember that Linda got the coat as a Christmas present from Santa. Rosine asked to try it on and when Linda handed it over to her, Rosine threw it on the ground and stomped on it saying it was, "a stupid coat, an ugly coat!" Time after time, she duped my sister into situations that inevitably ended in heartbreak. Rosine would treat Linda cruelly and later apologize, or she would treat Linda nicely and then later call her names. Rosine held out the promise of friendship, with a metaphorical knife up her sleeve.

....

I grew up in an age when the world looked forward to the future. Everything new was considered 'space-aged' and it seemed no harm could come to a society which was so technologically advanced. Surely our future would be easy, full of luxury, free time, and free of pain. And so it was for the first several years of my life. I had all I needed, I freely experimented with new ideas, time was my luxury, and substances, and I felt no pain. I picked up one long-lasting friend throughout those years. A friend who, through my own eyes, initially brought me social status and a sense of independence. A friend who went with me everywhere, every day, helping me to rebel and assert my adulthood. But my friend carried an even more lethal knife up her sleeve.

I remember sneaking my first cigarettes with a neighbor girl. She came from a 'rough' family and was a few years older than I. We would meet behind the semi-trucks at the gas station and puff away three or four cigarettes one after another iin rapid succession. It was a physical and psychological rush. Soon all the little girls in the neighborhood were trying out this sophisticated behavior. I took to it like I was born to smoke. Perhaps there was some truth to that. My father and grandfather were both smokers as were most adults in my life during the 1950s and 1960s. It was not a habit encouraged in children, but it was expected that all kids would try it at least once. My sister did just that. She tried it once and rejected it outright. I tried it once and was in love. I smoked walking to the bus stop, I smoked across the street from school, I smoked at football games and dances. It became part of my social persona. I remember watching two older, distant cousins smoking at a family reunion. I was so attracted to them. I thought they were the most worldly women I had ever seen and I longed for the day when I could be open about my smoking around family members.

Eventually independence and sophistication had nothing to do with my smoking. It simply degenerated into a nasty habit. I smoked within minutes of rising each morning and it was the last act I performed before bed each night. It was as natural as breathing...or so I told myself.

Over the years it took its toll. I developed a persistent cough and dark circles under my eyes. My adult voice grew deeper and raspier. Eventually I lost my teeth. I had cancer twice. And yet this insidious friend of mine would not let go. I was hypnotized, attended smoking aversion therapy, participated in smoking cessation programs, took numerous anti-smoking drugs, wore patches, chewed gum, and even had acupuncture. I quit more times than I could count. I can remember having quit one time and sitting in a Kmart parking lot bolstering my courage to go inside and get the things I needed without buying cigarettes. I sat in the car and cried for thirty minutes, trying to deny my need for my friend. In the end my craving for her overcame my desire to live without her.

With each failure to rid myself of cigarettes I lost more self-esteem and confidence. This relationship was no longer enjoyable for me, it made me feel weak, physically and spiritually. In the years since I began my relationship with tobacco, nearly everyone I knew had quit smoking. I looked at them and thought, "I'm as smart as he is," or "I'm as strong as she is." But with each successive failure I could no longer believe those statements. A part of me wanted to be weak and I hoped that I would be the one person in the universe that smoking did not kill. My friend robbed me of my ability to be rational and she kept duping me into the one situation that would inevitably end in heartbreak.

....

I remember my mother telling my sister, Linda, to just stand up to Rosine, to ignore her, or to find someone else to play with. To people who have never been in an obsessive relationship this advice sounds reasonable. But reason has little, if anything, to do with addiction.

BARGAINING

Paul Dominic Heckman

In *The Adventures of Tom Sawyer* by Mark Twain, Tom and two friends spend some time on Jackson Island in the Mississippi River. One night there is a terrifying storm, flashes of surreal lightning and cracking, roiling thunder torment Tom's soul and conscience. He spends the storm begging God to spare him from horrible, certain death. Tom promises to change his ways and to pray daily and attend church every Sunday. He bargains with the Supreme Being; he shakes and shivers and pleads for his life, if only God will give him one more chance. Then, frightened and exhausted, Tom drifts into sleep, fully intending to behave forever.

Day breaks clear and sunny, quiet and serene. Tom even wonders if the storm had been real. He is alive! Everything is all right and...and...normal. There was no need to worry. What was all that blubbering about? And before much time passes, Tom is again smoking and swearing and planning little tricks and crimes; HE is back to normal. What promises? And life goes on.

This type of human behavior is fairly common in the face of danger. We may ignore or doubt or take for granted that there is a God, but we hope there is no hell. I asked a doctor once why, even knowing the dangers, people continue to smoke. He simply said, "They always think they have time." And so we learn to bargain. "If this turns out all right I promise I'll never..." And when, in the short term, "this" turns out all right, many of us forget any deal. The point is that mortality will come sometime, in some way. If not now, later. To pin your hopes on being forgiven continuously and simply by paying dues to the club seems tenuous at best.

Rarely, if ever, do we think of what we are asking or even why we feel we have the right to ask. When our troubles come from our own choices and/or preventable dangers, the pleas seem selfish and hollow, though admittedly understandable. It's worth a shot. I'm not sure how I would respond in these situations if I were God.

Other dangers are unrelated to our choices or behaviors. Natural phenomena such as storms and droughts seem disconnected from our behaviors. In these situations, to plead for mercy is more respectable, though no more or less selfish. Again, if I were God I'm not sure what I would do.

And then there are those with an "I'm covered" attitude, which some people claiming religious piety seem to feel is sufficient no matter what. Simply saying, "I am a Christian", or "I am a Muslim", or "I am a Jew" does not excuse maladaptive behavior. This is selfishness and arrogance compounded by sanctimonious hypocrisy.

In these cases, if I were God, I would know exactly what I'd do. When the frightened bargainer awoke I would simply let the storm continue. If it is fear you need in order to live honestly and peacefully – it usually is arranged. But chosen consistency is always a good idea and you won't have to hope "there's time".

QUOTES

Above the cloud
with its shadow
is the star
with its light.
Victor Hugo

We are here to help each other.
Polar Eskimo saying

In the midst of winter,
I finally learned that there was in me
an invincible summer.
Albert Camus

Be kind,
everyone you know
is fighting a hard battle.
Philo of Alexandria 20BCE-40CE

If circumstances are bad
and you have to bear them
do not make them
a part of yourself.
paramahansa yogananda

Courage is resistance to fear,
mastery of fear –
not absence of fear.
Mark Twain

Fear knocked at the door.
Faith answered.
No one was there.
Old English legend

There are moments
in which one is
so completely alone.
Jules Renaud

FLORA'S TALE

Sara Slayton

(Based on Doug Lipman's work "Making Fairy Tales
from Personal Stories")

Once upon a time there lived a kindly old Queen who had long
ago given up hope that she would ever have a child. But one
day, as she walked along the river's edge she found a beautiful
Snowy Egret's egg. She wrapped it in her silk handkerchief and
gently placed it in the pocket of her ermine robe. She kept it
there for many long months until one day a lovely young
princess emerged. The Queen named her Flora because she was
born in the spring of the year and on her birth date the kingdom
sprang into bloom and the sun shone warmer than it ever had
before. At her christening all the people and gentle creatures
brought her flowers and other gifts, but the animals who loved
the dark were angry and many of them stayed away. Their
leader, the Great Grey Wolf was there and when he approached
the cradle he laid a dark cloth over the child's face and scratched
her with his sharp claws. Flora survived the attack but the Great
Gray Wolf was banished from the kingdom. He swore revenge
on the princess and she wore the scar of his anger on her little
cheek.

Every year Flora grew more charming and kind and she was beloved
by all. And each year, on her birthday, Flora and her mother went
to the river to thank the Snowy Egret for the gift of his egg. On the
day Flora turned 12 she went to the river as always but it seemed as
if the sun did not shine so brightly that day, she even saw some
wilted flowers, and most horribly she found the carcass of a rabbit
which had been savagely destroyed.

When she reached the river the Snowy Egret spoke to her. He
said, "Child, you will soon be the Queen, but there is a darkness

that is growing inside you. It was put there by the Great Gray Wolf and you must defeat him or you will not survive." "I can't do it!" she cried. "He is too fierce. I cannot defeat him." "You can and you must," replied the Egret. "Have courage child for you are stronger than you know." Flora trusted him completely so she agreed to do as he told her.

"You must go far to the north, for there the Wolf is building a kingdom of darkness and cold with which he will destroy you," said the Egret. "It is up to you to stop the growth of his domain. Take my fifty plume feathers and weave them into a robe for yourself. Each feather will hold my warmth to protect you from the cold where you must go. Use them when you need to light your spirit."

And so Flora plucked his feathers and wove them into a warm coat and she set off for the north country. She travelled for several days until she came to a strange meadow. Half of the meadow was bathed in sunlight, grasses and wildflowers bloomed, and the birds sang overhead. But the other half of the meadow was shrouded in a blanket of darkness, the ground was cold and barren, and there were no signs of life. The place made Flora tremble. She remained on the sunny side of the meadow, but that evening she watched the dark side. As the moon rose, the gloomy landscape was even more frightening and she could see shadowy figures moving in the distance. Then she heard it, the howl of the Great Grey Wolf. It took her breath away and her first instinct was to freeze where she stood. But she remembered the Snowy Egret's advice to have courage. Flora crept closer to the dark side, holding the feather coat close around her. In an instant, in total silence, two yellow eyes peered out at her – not more than an arm's length from her face. It was the Wolf. He snarled at her, showing his jagged teeth. Flora instinctively pulled the cloak over her face and as she did one of the plumes snapped in half. When it did, a spark

jumped from it. Quickly, she snapped another feather –
with the same result. Flora laid the feather coat on the
ground and grabbing great hands full of the feathers she
broke them as fast as she could. A flame leapt up and she
tossed the burning plumes onto the blanket of darkness.
Immediately it began to burn. She lifted up the corner of the
blanket and shook it. The fire spread. The Wolf tried to
extinguish the flames, but they spread too fast for him. He
gave one last terrifying howl and disappeared. Flora ran as
quickly as she could toward her home.

When she finally managed to get back to the river the Snowy
Egret was waiting for her. He smiled when he saw her
approach – glad that she had survived. Flora was filthy, and
tired, and weak. She fell at his feet and told him everything
that had happened. "You did well princess. But your work is
not done. The Great Wolf is very strong and you have only
wounded his pride. You must return and face him again." "I
can't do it!" she cried. "He is too fierce. I cannot defeat
him." "Have courage child," replied the Egret, "for you are
stronger than you know." Flora trusted him completely so
she agreed to do as he told her.

"You must return to the North and this time you must
wound the Great Wolf himself. Take my comb-claw as your
weapon." With that the Egret bit off the claw on his middle
toe and handed it to Flora. The comb was as sharp as steel.
But as the princess looked at the Egret she saw the pool of
bloody water around his feet. "You're hurt," she exclaimed.
"I no longer need the comb, my feathers are turning to
dust," he said. He looked weary and thin and Flora hugged
him before she left again.

This time she had to travel even farther because she had
driven the darkness back with her fire. By the time she

reached the edge of the gloom she was drained. She wondered how she would ever find the strength to face the Great Wolf. But this time, when the moon rose and he began to howl she did not freeze. Instead she watched him closely as he patrolled the edge of his inky kingdom. Back and forth, back and forth he paced. He seemed thinner, more frenzied. When the moon set he returned to his cave and fell into a fitful sleep. Flora watched him for two days and nights and always he did the same thing; howled at the moon, furtively loped along the edge of his realm, and then returned to the cave. On the third night she let him see her and although he could not cross the line between light and darkness he was very agitated. He barked and growled at her and chased her as she raced from one end of the dark line to the other. By the time the moon set the Great Wolf was exhausted. He returned to his cave to sleep. Flora waited until she heard his breathing grow deep. In silence she entered the cave. The den smelled of death and her head reeled at the odor. She drew the comb-claw and crept toward the Wolf. In one swift motion she grabbed his ear, lifted his head and drew the steely claw across his throat. The Wolf tried to scream, but Flora had cut his howl out of him. Flora ran as quickly as she could toward her home.

When she finally managed to get back to the river the Snowy Egret was waiting for her. He smiled when he saw her approach – glad that she had survived. Flora was filthy, and tired, and even weaker. She fell at his feet and told him everything that had happened. "You did well princess. But your work is not done. The Great Wolf is very strong and you have only wounded him. You must return and destroy him completely." "I can't do it!" she cried. "He is too fierce. I cannot defeat him." "Have courage child," replied the Egret, "for you are stronger than you know." Flora trusted him completely so she agreed to do as he told her.

"I have a very difficult thing I must ask you to do. Know that I ask it because it is your only hope." Flora saw that the Snowy

Egret looked haggard and gray, and that his remaining
feathers were turning to dust. "You must kill me child."
"Never!" she gasped, "I love you, I cannot kill you!" "But you
must or you will die," he responded. Although Flora trusted
him completely, this was too much to ask. "Please, there must
be some other way," she pleaded, but the Egret only shook his
head. "Use the comb-claw on me as you did on the Wolf and
after you kill me you must collect my blood in this vial. When
next you see the Wolf drink the vial. It will not harm you
much but it will be deadly to the Wolf."

"Please, no," she begged. "It is the only way," he maintained.
And finally because Flora trusted him completely she agreed
to do as he told her. Tearfully she cut across his slender white
neck, collecting his blood in the vial before he fell lifeless into
the river and floated away.

This time she had to travel even farther because she had
driven the Great Wolf back with her last attack. By the time
she reached his domain she could hardly stand because of her
weakness and her sorrow. She sat down in plain sight just on
the edge of the darkness and she waited until the moon rose.
As soon as she saw the Wolf's silhouette she drank the
contents of the flask. The liquid made her head reel and her
stomach churn, but she rose to her feet and stepped over the
dark line to face her enemy. As he drew nearer she could see
the scar across his throat. He was bone-thin and his eyes
were glazed. He could no longer howl, but only whimpered.
He sniffed at Flora detecting an acrid, dangerous scent. But
he was starving and desperate for revenge. With his last
ounce of strength he leapt at her throat and sank his teeth
into her soft flesh. They both fell to the ground, unconscious.

Flora awoke hours later with a searing pain in her neck. The ground around her was soaked with blood. The wolf lay dead a few feet away. Flora began the long walk home.

When she finally managed to get back to the river there was no one waiting for her, no welcome, no words of encouragement. She sat at the river's edge and began to cry. All her fear, all her pain, all her sorrow rained from her as her tears fell into the water. A familiar voice said, "You did well princess. Your work is done." Flora looked up into the eyes of a handsome prince, dressed all in white. He had a scar on his slender neck. It was her trusted advisor, the Snowy Egret. He lifted her to her feet, saying, "You are so brave and I love you." They were married and they ruled the kingdom with light, and warmth, and kindness for many years.

IS IT TIME?

Paul Dominic Heckman

Is it time? I won't complain; I just ask 'cause I feel sleepy.
Look at me; I have changed; there are so many things to
do now.
Why in the world, if it's time, does my list of work
get longer?
Can we stop, take a breath, hold each other?

I am sure, if it's time, that the sun will rise and set,
And when it does, this old world will keep on spinning.
So is it time for my shots? I'll hold my breath but
not forever;
We have a lot to do, and we'll do it when I'm better.

Is it time, to lie back down, insert the shields and
radiate me?
Does this mean we'll be done; I'll be home by noon?
How do you know that it's time, don't I have a say
in passing?
Can we stop, take a breath, hold each other?

I am sure, if it's time, that the moon will rise and shine,
And when it does you and I will keep on loving.
I'll hold still but don't take all day:
I've got things on my mind, and I really cannot stay.

Is it time, to take a look at all the causes of this demon?
Find a cure; find a way to crush its power?
How can it say when it's time? Aren't we stronger
than a mutant?
Can we stop, take a breath, hold each other?

I am sure, if it's time, while heaven waits for rhyme
and reason,
You and I will stop and breathe, and keep on holding.
So is it time? Lead the way; I will follow but please
be kind;
Is this the answer or the end? And I wonder: Is it time?

What is it now this time?
I wonder is it time?

From the musical play Until We Meet Again
By Sara M. Slayton and Paul D. Heckman

I'M GUESSING

Paul Dominic Heckman

If I should chance to talk with God some day,
And hear the music of His mighty voice,
I know that I would ask why men decay,
And plead to make, once more, another choice.

Before our birth and after death we're caught,
The curse of being born as mortal men.
In darkness deep we lie without a thought,
The sights and sounds within us lost again.

For Life's eternal wisdom is cut short
By Death's cold, heartless drive on men to reign,
And lies to all upon this earthly fort
That knowledge here foregoes the mortal pain.

'Tisn't true, God," I'd say then much bolder,
"Death does not please more than growing older."

CANCER LOGIC

Sara Slayton

"How did it happen?"

"I was dancing."

"When did it happen?"

"At ten this morning."

Now I've got her attention. She looks up at me and pictures some sort of lunatic in leotards prancing through a maze of office cubicles. I'll let her make her own picture; it's easier on both of us.

"Who's your regular doctor?"

Now how do I answer this question? Do I tell her I've had cancer twice in my life so I'm pretty damned close to the oncologist, or do I just give her the name of my GYN? Well, this is a minor thing; I decide I can keep the cancer man out of the loop this time. "Her name is Margaret, from the Women's Health Center."

"OK. Now we just have to get you registered and then a doctor will see you. Let me wheel you over to Lucy."

Lucy, who is half my age, is wearing thick-soled shoes and a long denim skirt that swishes when she moves. I made one like it in college from an old pair of jeans.

"How did it happen?"

"I was dancing."

"When did it happen?"

"At ten this morning."

"Did it happen at work?"

This is a loaded question. If it happened at work my insurance company may make a workers' comp stink. I say, "Yes, it happened in the building where I work," adding, 'but it truly was all my own fault. You see, I was trying to teach a bunch of people who will be teachers how to tap dance with kids. You tape some washers onto the soles of your shoes and it sounds just like taps." She doesn't write that all down, but it's not lost on her that I chose to dance at work this morning.

She makes a wristband for me. It has an orange tab. I think how my grandson would like it. Orange is his favorite color right now. I make a lame attempt to engage Lucy and to distract myself from a rising rush of terror. "Now I can swim all day?" The remark only convinces her that the dancing lady is a nut case.

"You can wait out here," she says as she pushes me gently into the hallway.

My husband is there, sitting, or more accurately bouncing in a chrome and foam cushion chair...orange again I note. Now the full flush of panic is on us both. We recognize this hallway and the examining rooms beyond it. We know this is only a slight injury, but it was only a small pain last time. A fire ball of fear is rising up in me. When it gets to my mouth it instantly becomes tears and a quiet moan. As I look down at the floor I can see my husband's leg jumping, as if he's listening to some driving punk song in his head. More probably his leg is simply mimicking his rising blood pressure and pulse. We recognize what's happening, even comment on it ever so slightly and then we stop talking because we can't say any more with the feeling upon us. Panic sucks our breath away.

We can't do this together. There's a sense that this is all so trivial, but I also feel a need to do something differently from the last time...anything that might break the pattern.

"Go home," I tell him, "I'll be fine. No sense you sticking around here. You know how long this all takes." I'm trying to sound as cavalier as I can. He takes the lure of escape and fresh air, knowing as well as I do that we have to change these circumstances.

He is my rock. Without him I cannot face anything serious. If he leaves I know that I will be all right. This is the crazy logic that cancer breeds.

MS. TRAUMA

Sara Slayton

My fifth grade gym teacher had dark hair on his hands and a shaved head that sported a distinct black shadow. A short man, with a strong build, he was formidable to me and every other one of my gawky, jug-eared peers. He was only my second male teacher and I was intimidated by his obvious masculinity. His voice was deep and would echo off the walls of our little gym. There was a heat that came off his body and he often glistened with sweat. In addition to being an imposing figure, he was also diabolical and liked the fear he saw in our eyes as we lined up in bony-kneed rows. It became evident that the more fear a child displayed, the more likely she was to induce, and have to deal with, his sinister nature.

I went all through school with a dove-like girl named Marla. She was soft in all ways - in manner, in physical appearance, and in her speech. She had a slight speech anomaly that made her pronounce the "ch" sound as "sh". She went to speech therapy once a week and I think she was somewhat embarrassed at being singled out in this way. She was pale-skinned and reddened easily. We all knew her to be an agreeable and humble classmate.

The gym teacher sniffed out Marla's vulnerability almost immediately. He would call her to the front of the gym and make her pronounce words such as "chair" and "chicken". She would do it as he looked on with a reptilian air. Having this kind of power to humiliate Marla, and all the rest of us, exhilarated him.

After fifth grade I never again heard Marla mispronounce a "ch" word. Between speech therapy and the gym teacher's relentless humiliation, she learned to overcome the softness of her enunciation. But she did so at the expense of her gentle nature.

....

I remember being at a house party about a year after my first battle with cancer. Hardly anyone there knew about my illness. Most of them met me when I was in remission and accepted my short hair as a fashion choice. It was rather nice to have a group of people who didn't share that part of my history, because they didn't know to ask how I was feeling and coping with my new life. At one point I went into the kitchen to get a beer from the refrigerator. There were two people sitting at the table kicking around some ideas about how people learn. As an educator, I have always enjoyed this discussion and I listened in as I searched for a bottle opener. The woman was arguing the merits of trauma as a teacher. She believed that traumatic events, although unpleasant, were indeed powerful teachers. She even went so far as to postulate that for some people trauma was maybe the only, and therefore best, teacher. Her theory was that living through negative experiences would motivate a person and set her on the "right path".

Without warning, to myself or anyone else I began to hiss like the beer I was opening. I attacked her flimsy argument with a fury that no one expected. I explained to her that only someone who had never had to face trauma could be so cold in her assessment of its merits. I was furious with her offhand dismissal of another person's pain and anguish. I chided her for her lack of humanity and for her superior demeanor. I attacked her argument in a fury of animated heat. When I felt the sweat come creeping along my hairline I recognized my own rage and stopped. The word 'lunatic' hung heavily in the room as I set my bottle down and walked out the back door.

In a moment of fantasy I turned back to the woman and said, "How's that for a traumatic lesson?" as the screen door slapped shut behind me. It was a satisfactorily dramatic illusion.

....

Many times since that night I have asked myself what I learned from my own personal sessions with trauma. Had I changed my lifestyle? Not in any substantial ways. I was never like the survivors in the magazines who turned their lives around after a bout with cancer. Those women proudly kept their hair short, ran two miles a day, and ate only organic and macrobiotic foods. I returned to nearly the same life I had before my diagnosis and treatment. The 'right path' argument fell pretty flat with me.

What trauma taught me was the same thing Marla learned from our gym teacher; that to be soft and innocent seemed to invite the hard lessons. The choice then was to become hardened and to carry on, try to anticipate the lessons, and to identify early on those who would teach them to us. I'm not sure about Marla, but for me the lesson had the bitter taste of loss and sorrow.

FACED WITH THE PROSPECT

Paul Dominic Heckman

Honey, sit down, I've got something to tell you.

Her son, eleven year old Ryan sat on the back porch with
nothing to do. Lost, he stared through the screen into the
dusk, his gaze fixed on a dim yard light which grew brighter as
evening fell. His stare caused peripheral images to fade in and
out of focus; the barn became a dark mass with no distinct
features, and then reappeared as, obviously, the barn. Bushes
and shrubbery drifted into smokish blurs and returned to
distinct shapes. When he looked away from the light bulb,
Ryan traced the ghosting image of light across the yard.
Blinking a few times and adjusting to the lesser light of the
western sky, he sighed heavily. For Ryan, reality was
uncertain; unable to control his helplessness, he dreamt of
magic.

...so they want to be sure it hasn't spread.

If only things could disappear and reappear as something else.
If my school could vanish and come back as a starship, I could
be in charge. I could say what's what and disappear anything I
wanted. He went on for some time envisioning himself
returning from space – the unknown - his starship humming
over the hills above his home. The ship would be so big and
powerful it would take an hour just to pass over his town. I'd
need the whole city to land on...at the fairgrounds! Everybody
would see me! And my Mom!

Well, it means cancer.

There was a faint and sudden smack of sound from the yard.
Ryan alerted and scanned the field from his command post,
adjusting his eyes to the dull pulse of light from the bulb. Gnats
swarmed erratically in a lump around the cone of light released

from under thelamp cover. He noticed them because of their sheer mass. He stood and walked to the porch door, stepping out onto the well-worn gravel path that led to the barn. The screen door slapped shut as only screen doors do, and Ryan walked toward the light. He was cautious as both sharp and dull obstacles pressured his probing bare feet along the way.

Well, uh, there's gramma on your dad's side, and my cousin, aunt Denise...and...

At the base of the lamp pole Ryan saw the caramel-colored undercarriage of a June bug's bulky misfortune. He crouched and gently righted the insect. He had seen thousands of these lumbering bugs; they were harmless. All they ever did was bump into things and land helplessly on their backs. The bug clicked its wings, reassembled them to the appearance of a shiny maroon shell, and tumbled off through the wet grass with flustered indignity. There were no thanks.

I know; thank you, honey. I'm going to be all right.

The dark mass of gnats hovering above him descended to his shoulders. Despite their seemingly unpredictable patterns they remained several inches from his face. Then, because his head offered them nothing, the insects, en masse, shifted back to the bulb above. God, he thought, why would God make such a thing?

Sometimes chills. Sometimes fever.

By now the dampness of the night air had floated into the yard. It was the humid heaviness before storms, and Ryan's feet were wet from the sweating lawn. He returned to the porch and sighed at the total lack of direction the evening was taking. A fog was sliding in across the fields. It was thick, making it impossible to tell what lay in the distance.

He slumped into his chair just as a blanket flash of heat lightning framed the horizon. It was too distant to affect his immediate surroundings, but he had a sense of what was coming. Another flash burnished the distant hills in a brilliant, spectral flare.

Radiation and chemo, I suppose...

Prepare for warp speed! Engines, fire! Star base Cassandra, come in! Again a flash, much closer, exploded and the barn and foliage were frosted cold-blue from the powerful Starship's thrust. Thundering news echoed among the out buildings. The yard light became insignificant, a dim retreating planet, as Ryan charged toward the unknown with all the bravery of not knowing.

Alien fleet approaching! Engage protector shields! Explosive charges battered the ship. Radiation proton beams, fire! His science was uncertain. The air held the rich smells of a coming storm. Ryan knew enough to assume victory. He knew the big words. X-ray! Stenosis stable! Fire all CCs! FLASH! We need... KKKEEERRACK! We're hit, we're hit! FLASH! Engine room... KKKEEERRACK! We're being overrun. We're being boarded! Cassandra! Do you read me? Cassandra, do you know me? Communication was unclear, questionable. Blinding sheets hid clarity. Words thundered! Ryan slammed his chair from side to side. The assault was a barrage of cascading, dense explosions, battering the command post – the sanctum of Ryan's control and understanding. Another FLASH held life suspended; time froze in the deep cold blue...four seconds and a lifetime were the same. Ryan leaned forward, swinging his focus to the port scanner of the bridge. What the...?

The truth took a moment to register. There, somehow inside

the porch, just inches from his face, clutching the screen, frozen, powerful, and terrifying, was a massive Luna moth! EEEYOW! Holy Shit! God! Jesus! Ryan invoked the learned response to danger and fell back into his seat. Another flash of lightning defined the revelation. He lunged forward. A friggin' moth! A Luna moth! It shifted its stout body, more from the onslaught of rain than from Ryan's outburst. Its body was easily two inches in length; its front wings spread three inches on either side, and the hind wing projections made it almost six inches in length.

They say if it's not growing, maybe we can wait...we may not have to do anything right away.

Against the light from the yard and the occasional lightning flashes, the moth was outlined in white; its shadow completely covering Ryan's face. For several moments both Ryan and the moth remained securely fastened to their perches. The moth's antennae twitched occasionally, and Ryan blinked once or twice. Major motion was confined to the small blocks of rain in the grid of the screen that would hold anxiously and then burst in rivulets onto the sill below.

The MRI shows one long streak...we'll have to see.

After a time Ryan wiped the moisture from his eyes; the moth shuddered in the mist of a rain subsiding, and rumbling thunder weakened, announcing its hour had passed. Ryan raised his hand to the moth. Its wings, with yellow rings, remained stationary until Ryan's fingers brushed the web of screen to which the moth held fast. It shuddered. Ryan jerked back his hand. I won't hurt you.

Don't be scared, honey. It's going to be all right.

The moth seemed to clutch the screen more tightly. In the dimness of the limited light, the strange mass seemed regal and powerful. "I won't hurt you," Ryan repeated. He reached toward the moth. "What are you, huh? You just trying to stay outta sight?" He gently ran his fingers along the body. The moth twitched and pushed away from the screen. Ryan's hand fell away as the moth hefted itself, fluttered, beat against the screen several times, and resettled a few inches away.

Really, they know what they're doing.

I never saw anything like you before in real life. Where you from, huh? You just wanna hide here from the rain? Ryan chuckled nervously. I thought you were an alien, really! I was just thinking about a space attack and 'BAM' you were right there. I mean nobody ever thinks that an alien is gonna be right there, you know? Ryan examined the moth. He leaned in close to the screen and saw small vibrations; he though he heard a low hum. Ryan glanced around the porch and noticed an empty fruit jar on a nearby table. He calmly stood to retrieve it.

It won't take long; they'll see what needs to be done to get my life back on track.

I'm just going over here, he said and lifted the jar, slowly unscrewing the lid. Returning to the screen, he was sure he could hear the rhythmic humming and see the vibration of the moth's immediate life.

Do you want to be free, huh? You wanna live outside? The moth scuttled up the screen. Ryan raised the jar. You wanna be outta here, huh? Just inches away, Ryan centered the mouth of the jar over the moth and pushed. The moth flapped wildly into the jar to escape and Ryan pulled back to clamp on the lid. Well, tough, he finished.

So it shouldn't take long. We'll see what's what and do what we have to do.

Ryan sat back in his chair and grinned. He shook the jar
violently several times, listening to the dull thud of the insect
as it slammed from side to side. Finally, Ryan held the jar still
and peered closely at the strange thing he had captured. The
moth lay at the bottom, its curled body barely moving.
Moisture appeared on the inside of the jar and Ryan held it
up against the light of the yard lamp. If you were an alien,
you'd have to do more than just scare the shit out of me.

The doctors say we can beat this.

Ryan stood and carried the jar to the bathroom, pulling the
light chain above the sink as he entered. He sat on the edge
of the tub facing the toilet. Again he shook the jar, taking an
unusual pleasure from the sound. The jar was steamy inside
and lines of moisture trickled down its sides. The moth's
wings were stuck together as it lay, only breathing, in the
dampness of the bottom.

No, it won't be as scary as last time.

Ryan unscrewed the lid. Immediately he smelled a strange
chemical smell, a mustiness, and felt a slight warmth rise
from the opening. The moth did not move, Ryan tried
squeezing his hand into the jar. It wouldn't fit. He looked
about for something to pry the ugly lump from the bottom.
There was nothing he could immediately recognize as
appropriate. Finally, he tipped the jar over his left hand. At
first only moisture rolled from the lip and ran between his
fingers.

...because it's hard to know if you've got a hold of it all.

Come on, I want you outta there. He tapped the jar against
the palm of his hand. The moth slid a little way down the
side. He tapped again. Now, the wings of the moth were

outside the rim, though the body still held in the moisture. Ryan placed the jar at his feet. He wiped his hands on his pants and reached for the wings. He peeled the moth from the mouth of its cage and held it up to the light. The full power of its wings was gone, but what little remained was evident; this had been a strong creature.

Of course, I'll need you to take care of things here.

Thought you were gonna be free didn't you? The moth shivered its remaining strength and twitched its wings in Ryan's hand. Ryan yelped and threw it down hard on the tile floor.

He composed himself and retrieved the moth, shaking it violently. You're pretty tough, you know that? He held the limp insect over the toilet bowl. The glare of porcelain framed Ryan's hand and the moth for only an instant. When it finally stopped bobbing and the water became still, Ryan could see the faint movement of labored breathing along the beast's sleek abdomen. There was no humming, he was sure.

Now don't worry...we're gonna beat this.

Suddenly, Ryan was watching the gushing water swirl in a counter-clockwise manner. He absently recalled that in the southern hemisphere, toilets flush in a clock-wise manner. To a creature in a whirlpool it doesn't make any difference.

I love you, honey, and I'll be home soon.

Ryan watched the moth spin violently in the gushing downpour; the suction noise echoed in the bowl and subsided. As he walked out to the porch he didn't notice immediately that the gnats had regrouped about the yard light and a June bug was hitting itself on the barn wall. The storm had moved on to another distance. And though Ryan would again be in control someday, for now he surveyed the damage of the attack and stared through the wavy lines of moisture that held anxiously before slipping into rivulets and dropping to the sill below.

TIDES
Sara Slayton

The first time I saw the Atlantic Ocean I was nine years old.
My father packed up the family plus an old maiden aunt and
we headed for St. Petersburg, Florida. We were going to visit
some obscure relatives there. I was thrilled with the prospect
of spending weeks on the beach running around in the Florida
sunshine. It was everything I expected. My skin turned nut-
brown as I raced up and down the shoreline in front of our
little housekeeping cabin. Each morning I got up early to
meet the man who ran the resort as he went out to feed the
seagulls. He would bring a bag of leftover bread which we
would toss up as the gulls sailed in over our heads to pick it
out of the air. It was thrilling and their screeches made me
believe they were thankful. I would spend the next hour or so
walking along the water line collecting sea shells. The tide left
an odd assortment of strange and twisted shells, along with
many things I did not recognize. I was a midwestern kid who
knew nothing about marine life. The receding tide often left
bits of skeletons and plant life that were entirely foreign to
me. I would sit and contemplate the creatures from which
this flotsam had come. It made the ocean a place of great
mystery and intrigue. I believed in its power and life-giving
essence.

....

The first time I had cancer my husband, and two sons, and I
headed for the ocean the day after my last radiation
treatment. Again, it was all I hoped for and Daytona Beach
proved to be my cure. One morning I got up before the boys,
got a cup of coffee and went out to the beach. There I made a
little nest for myself. From that warm vantage point I sipped
my coffee and watched the gulls soaring and landing. It was
there that I first let myself accept the possibility that I was

going to get well.

The night before I had eaten meat for the first time in over half a year. A leftover piece of steak on my son's plate had actually looked good to me and when I put it in my mouth it tasted rich and hearty. The metallic chemo residue that had coated my tongue for months seemed to have faded. Now, the aroma and taste of my morning coffee was rich, too, as it hadn't been for so long. I knew these were good signs. They were things the doctors had told me to "look forward to."

My hair began to grow back about a month before we went to the beach. I was still wearing a wig most of the time, but in the ocean I liked the rush of salt water over my nearly bald skull. It was like a weird sort of skinny-dipping. I wondered what my hair would be like. So many people had told me that it would be curly or red. That kind of thing is known as 'cancer folklore'. Such stories are spread by healthy people who have known someone who has gone through this terrible mess. In their naiveté they believe one cancer is like the next. It's similar to the way people tell pregnant women all those horror stories about labor.

....

Thirteen years later, my husband and I returned to Daytona Beach. I had a nagging pain in my gut that I was trying to ignore, or explain away as a result of eating too much fast food and sitting in the car for hours on end. We rented a little cabin right on the beach from which I could hear the tide all night long. It was November, and this time there was grayness to it all that I couldn't overlook. The wind had a bite to it and the water was too cold for swimming. However, I was content to spend my days walking, searching for shells and listening to the gulls screech. I remembered that when I was a girl I had scraped knees from playing recklessly and hard. My father told me that the ocean would heal those sores, but that there would be a bit of a price to pay. He was right. The salt water stung my legs, but in a few days the sores were clean and healed.

Maybe it would have been different if I could have gone swimming that November. As it was, when I returned home I found that my cancer had returned and that the prescribed treatment would heal me, but at a very nasty price. I would have much preferred the sunny, salt water cure of Daytona.

DR. DE-I-ETY

Paul Dominic Heckman

Folks, clear the way;
Step aside for the man who can work miracles,
And he has!

Show some respect for the man in the suit
Who gives cancer the boot;
Let him pass.
It's a miracle! And there ain't no doubt,
We're all here to serve,
And on call to shout:

[Refrain]
Doctor D! Doctor D! Doctor De-i-ety
Hand him your X-rays, and count on your next days
'cause he is the one, count on him son,
to get the job done.

Soon, with heavenly grace, like a hand from above,
He pulls on a glove, and he grins.
Shine glorious light, steal the dark from the night,
Everything is all right – let's begin.

Standing tall and bold, like the Man upstairs,
You have got to know – He's the one who spares.

[Refrain]
Doctor D! Doctor D! Doctor De-i-ety
Hand him your X-rays, and count on your next days,
'cause he is the one, count on him son,
to get the job done.

"What we got here is an evil beast,
And when I look in its face
My wrath is unleashed, 'cause that's how I operate.
And if that evil spreads, I just gather my will
And nod my sweet head,
'cause that's how I operate."

Ask the nurses now, they will always say, "cause His heart is
pure, he will save the day."

From the musical play Until We Meet Again
by Sara M. Slayton and Paul D. Heckman

DISTRACTIONS AND THE DISCONNECT
Paul Dominic Heckman

People behave in subconscious proportion to their ability to cope with the knowledge of their own mortality. It is an irksome and confusing process but what primarily sets us apart from other living things. Nature follows its course; people seek distractions.

From the coast of Massachusetts, a forest-green mansion overlooks the Atlantic. Under the many green and white awnings of the first floor windows, shrubbery surrounds the estate. The lawn is meticulously cultivated, sculpted, and growing in lush patterns of walkways and gardens. At the base of the sloping yard, a white band of warm sand is hidden or revealed with the tides; narrowing and widening with the bends of the sun and the moon.

On a day warm and clear, sea breezes kiss the curves of stranded ocean creatures on shore, and a seemingly one-way slap onto land is resolved with a ticket from the sun that thrusts them back into Neptune's bulging cradle. Back and forth the process volleys, a rhythm too fine for many human ears.

From their lounge chairs by the pool, Agnes and Charles stare at a mist they have made in their eyes.

"I can't believe she's gone."

A clam is showered with spray and somersaults back into the sea.

"It seems so empty now."

Ridges in the sand reshape to spell waterwords in the kamikaze language of the stars.

Agnes turns to Charles. She is tall, even while sitting, but her shoulders slump with invisible weight. Charles breathes heavily, unevenly, and low.

"She didn't leave a will, that's what gets me."

"Will we have to sell...?"

Dolphins break the blue line. Their sounds disperse long before land. From the house the radio spits tin and Agnes snaps. The air is full of choices.

"Maybe one of the cars...the boat..."

"I'll miss..."

The sun takes a breather and the ocean falls silent. Below in the depths weights settle by size. Feeders find this natural. It is.

"I'll have to keep working, that's for sure."

"Can we pay the taxes?"

"There's probably some way around that."

Driftwood tickles algae in a gentle ebb. Sea fronds fold out and wiggle to an eddy.

"Wanna' play some tennis?"

"What?"

"Tennis?"

"Why not?" For years they had kept score.

Charles and Agnes walked hand and hand to the court. Agnes beat Charles 6-4, 6-2, 6-4. Once again they were pretty much even.

COVERAGE
Paul Dominic Heckman

Progress should occur with an eye on humanity and never at the expense of true choice. When rules make the world perfect, what manner of life will embrace it?

A few years ago Nickleby Wheeler, the youngest child in a working-poor family, watched her father dying. Summer heat drew life from him like oil wells suck from the earth. In his wall-papered bedroom her father lay in the moistness of his knowledge. Nickleby, who was twelve, sat by his side and listened.

"...Viet Nam was hot like this" he rasped, "hot and fighting," he coughed "...freedom...," he wheezed.

Nickleby looked away toward the compendium of objects on her father's dresser. The possessions that surrounded her were these: an empty wallet, a clock, a watch, a desk calendar, three prescription bottles, an empty potato chip bag, a Saint Christopher statue, a radio, a small TV, and a file of papers labeled Important Papers (titles, income taxes 1986-2006), and several insurance policies wrapped tightly in dry and flimsy rubber bands.

In her mind Nickleby saw the life of a man reduced to a stack of pulp, tin, and faith, the accumulated wealth of a poor man fooled by convention and convenience, all the while feeding him air-blown carbohydrates and keeping him dancing to a digital knell. He was dying, she thought, in a hothouse of department store props. Everyone dies, she thought, but someone else tells you what to leave behind. Measures of time, and papers of authority, and newsy entertainment were the proof and reassurance that his life had been played by the earthly rules and he would now move on, bought and paid for, covered and secure, for the heavenly set of rules above.

The sun bossed its way through the bedroom's west window. The heavy air creased the man's body like a steam press as he clutched his chest where a soul just might be.

Nickleby absently reached to the stack of policies (loopholes?) In the mind of a child; negotiable limits and 'pre-existing condition' certificates in the minds of investors – mortality IS a pre-existing condition!) and the rotted restraints snapped; papers shuffled and sifted to the floor. The policies were up to date, she would find out later, but would also prove to be insufficient. She left the room and naturally called her older brother before anyone else.

A doctor from the hospital told her later that her father might have lived had she called an ambulance first. "She didn't," her brother said, "because his coverage was denied and the family couldn't afford it."

"My God! That's putting a price on human life!" the doctor said.

"Yes. Isn't it?" he replied

MEA CULPA
Sara Slayton

...to all who have to work harder
    Because I can't work at all,
...to all who have to carry heavier burdens
    Because I have a weight-lifting restriction,
...to all who are tired
    Because I can only sleep,
...to all who are holding me up
    Because my arms are weak,
...to all who are standing behind me
    Because I can't turn my head to see you.
...to all who resent my rare social invitation
    Because it doesn't include them.
...to all whose scheduled lives have been interrupted
    Because I can't predict my future,
...to all who have to go out of their way
    Because I have lost mine,
...to all who have wished me well
    Because I don't get better,

I am sorry, I am sorry, I am truly sorry.

You may think I have made some poor choices, and you
wouldn't be wrong, but never in my wildest dreams
would I have chosen this particular nightmare to hurt you.

So be it....

"UNTIL WE MEET AGAIN"
a musical play in two acts

Scene Summary

Set Design   67
Cast   68
Narrator: Prologue   69
Scene 1: Radiation Waiting Room   71
       Song: Is It Time?   74
Scene 2: Radiation Marking   78
Scene 3: Meet Suddards & Jackie   83
       Song: That Makes Me A Freak   90
Scene 4: Dr. Deity and Dr. Franco   91
       Songs: Dr. Deity   92
       Tropical Cancer   97
Scene 5: Mr. Probowski's Daughter   99
Scene 6: Radiation Waiting Room   101
       Song: Darling Of The Waiting Room   105

Intermission

Act 2:
Scene 1: Coffee Shop   108
       Song: If You Need Anything, Just Ask   112
Scene 2: Suddards' Post Op   114
Scene 3: Boomer's Question   119
       Song: Boomer's Got A Question   125
Scene 4: Suddards' Hospice   126
       Song: (reprise) That Makes Me A Freak   130
Scene 5: Doctors and Gods   131
       Song: Hush Now   132
Scene 6: Passing The Torch   133
       Song: (reprise) Darling Of The Waiting Room   134

Basic Set Design:

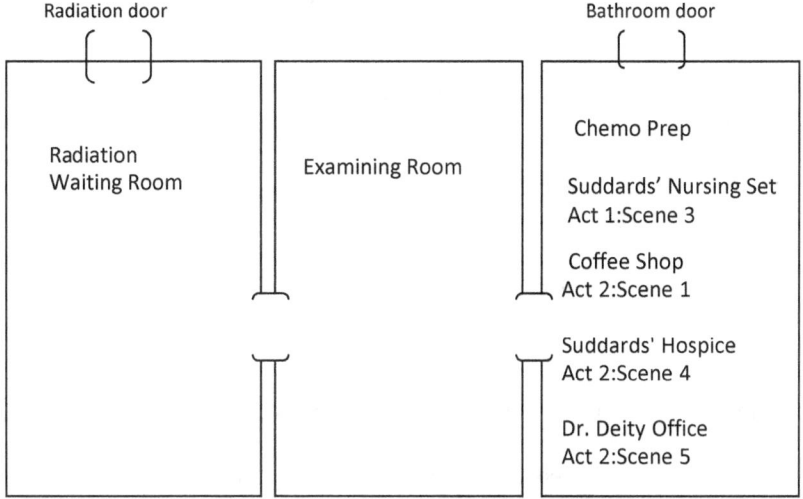

Notes:

Darling uses the Radiation Waiting Room, Suddards uses the Chemo Prep. They both use the Examining Room, but never meet...each staying to either the left or right of the stage.

The Examining Room has 3 large, X-ray type panels along the back of it onto which different images are projected throughout the play.

There are parallel doors in the Examining Room which lead to the Radiation Room or the Chemo Prep Room.

Cast:

Darling: attractive woman in her mid-thirties, bald, has non-hodgkin's lymphoma in her throat

Suddards: large man in his late sixties, pancreatic cancer, dramatically loses weight as the play progresses

Bernith: (prounced ber-neeth) 74 year old, widowed farm wife, treatable cancer of some sort

Mr. Probowski: 92 year old, retired math teacher, brain cancer, first to die; red hair - goes bald

Wally: 70 year old, prostate cancer

Rueben: 75 year old, lung cancer

Boomer: 58 year old, ex-hippie, testicular cancer

Dr. Deity: sophisticated, salt & pepper hair, mid-fifties, wears expensive suit

Dr. Franco: Dr. Deity's resident, rushed, sleep-deprived, late twenties

Jackie: male nurse, in his thirties

Nurse: Any age female

Cyan: coffee shop customer, mid to late thirties, friend of Darling.

Mary Catherine: coffee shop customer, late twenties, friend of Darling, large woman, fairly bold personality wearing a cross necklace.
Dual role = Volunteer Act 1

Mona: coffee shop customer, thirties, friend of Darling, thin, nervous.
Dual Role = Volunteer Act 2;Scenes 3 & 6

Nancy : Mr. Probowski's daughter, has long then short red hair.
Dual role = Intern Act 2; Scenes 2 & 4 (not red hair)

Mother: young woman.
Dual roles = Coffee Shop Waitress & Intern Act 1 Scene 3; Act 2; Scene 4

Child: female, around eight years old

Prologue: [Darling: taped audio. Black & white photographs of girls and boys in "western wear" are projected]

When I was a little girl, my friends and I would often put on a "show". We would gather together the usual bunch of reluctant volunteers- younger siblings, moms, pets - as our captive audience. Often, we had the bravado to charge admission to these little bits of amusement; maybe a penny or a piece of candy. In elaborate pieces of cos-tume, we would share our dubious talents until the dogs wandered off, with the toddlers shortly behind them. Eventually the faithful mothers, who had to get back to the serious business of the day, would clap politely. This was our signal to wind things up.

We staged many of these neighborhood productions in a summer's time. We danced in oversized high heels, we did magic tricks with props purchased from the Woolworth's store, we sang silly songs in plucky, if not tuneful, voices and we often dressed up our dogs and cats - accepting the applause for their tricks.

We imagined ourselves to be legends in our own time and dreamed of illustrious futures. In those days we yearned for the ability to see who we would become and to know what adventures awaited us. In our mind's eyes we became famous, but kindly, champions. We were certain that our futures would be full of chivalrous and daring deeds. No one among us imagined the likelihood of illness, nor did we have a frame of reference in which to place such a concept. We knew someday we would grow old and die, but that was a vaporous notion at best.

My greatest hope and ambition as a child was to become a cowgirl. It was the age of TV westerns and I was charmed by every detail of the genre. I liked the clothes; I loved the horses, and the appeal of a maverick attitude was potent. I was sure I would become the kindly rancher's steely-eyed daughter, who would rescue animals and eat beans from a tin plate. Not only did I believe this was possible, I had faith that it was probable.

I took this vision with me everywhere and when it was my turn to take the stage I did so as the rancher's daughter. I stood behind the blanket we had hung across the garage door in tooled, leather-look boots and wearing a fringed vest I had made from a brown bag. I would saunter out to center stage and croon my favorite anthem, "Happy Trails To You", often adding a few whoops and hollers to under-score my character.

Never once did I imagine the trail's end.

Act One:
Scene 1: The Radiation Waiting Room

[Dark stage. Eerie glow and hum come from under the heavy metal door upstage]

VOICE: Breathe...Don't breathe...*[whirring sound]*...Breathe

[Spot comes up on Darling sitting in a utilitarian chair. She looks vacantly from left to right.]

[Spot draws back illuminating the entire stage, revealing a radiation waiting room. There are utilitarian chairs, a few tables (one with a jigsaw puzzle on it), a coffee cart, some magazines, a toy box full of toys, an aquarium, a bulletin board and there is a large plant on an end table...as the play progresses it loses more leaves.]

[There is a sign saying "ONCOLOGY" in the room. At the back of the set is a heavy metal door with radiation - danger signs on it.]

[Bernith, Wally and Rueben are seated. They are in different states of awareness and recognition...staring off and down, Bernith is turning pages of a magazine.]

[The volunteer enters; puts a poster on the bulletin board "Living With Cancer Workshop" then makes coffee, feeds fish, waters plant.]

[Darling looks at each person.]

[Mr. Probowski enters in wheelchair, pushed by Nancy]

NANCY: Oh, dear, are we late?

RUEBEN: No, no, don't worry. They haven't called anyone in yet. They're running a little behind.

NANCY: Thank God. I have such a struggle getting dad's chair out of the van.

MR. PROBOWSKI: Ya, I'm a real pain these days.

NANCY: It's not you dad, it's just this silly chair. It's so heavy and awkward. I'm always afraid I'm going to leave it unlocked and then just dump you right out of it.

MR. PROBOWSKI: Yeah, we wouldn't want me jeopardizing my health. *[laughs]*

RUEBEN: Yeah, falling down...ouch! *[laughs]*

WALLY: My ma was in a wheelchair when I was a little boy. It was wicker with a leather seat ...creaked just like an old saddle.

RUEBEN: Ya, I remember the kind.

WALLY: She died when I was 9, but we had that chair around for years after.

NANCY: Dad, you stay put. I'm going to move the van. I'll be right back.

[NANCY exits]

MR. PROBOWSKI: Where would I go?

WALLY: I wonder whatever happened to that old chair...and my Ma *[touching/admiring Mr. P's wheelchair]*

RUEBEN: Well, this is no time to worry about it...too late now.

MR. PROBOWSKI: God knows where stuff gets to. I spent half of yesterday looking for my clothes brush. After church, when I took off my suit, I noticed all this hair on my jacket. And do you think I could find that brush? Nowhere!

RUEBEN: Do people still use those things?

MR. PROBOWSKI: I hadn't used it in years. I can't imagine where it's got to. But I need it, my hair is...all over my good suit. I want to look good.

RUEBEN: What difference does it make now? People don't look at us or if they do all they see is sick.

[They all go back to reading/looking around]

[Nurse enters]

NURSE: Mr. Probowski? *[No answer]*

NURSE: Mr. Probowski?

[Everyone looks at Mr. Probowski]

[Nurse goes to Mr. Probowski and touches his hand]

MR. PROBOWSKI: Is it time? Where's my daughter?

NURSE: We're ready to start. Your daughter will know where you are.

MR. PROBOWSKI: It's my time?

[Nurse steers Mr. Probowski to the metal door...consoling, assisting. She opens the door.]

[Mr. Probowski stops, turns back to others.]

MR. PROBOWSKI: I guess it's time...tell my daughter *[Nurse and Mr. Probowski exit through the metal door.]*

SONG: Verses 1 & 2 of "Is It Time?"
Lyrics by Paul Heckman
Music by Hans Mayer

[Sung by Bernith]
Is it time? I won't complain,
I just ask 'cause I feel sleepy
Look at me; I have changed;
There are so many things to do now.
Why in the world, if it's time,
Does my list of work get longer?
Can we stop, take a breath, hold each other?

[Sung by Wally & Rueben]
I am sure, if it's time,
That the sun will rise and set
And when it does, this old world
Will keep on spinning.
So is it time for my shots?
I'll hold still but not forever;
We have a lot to do
And we'll do it when we're better.

[Wally and Rueben go back to staring and Bernith starts turning magazine pages again. Darling looks at the door and at each of the other three people.]

BERNITH: He guesses it's time. *[Pause]*

[Old folks recognize that Darling is much younger...they look at her as she looks down. Bernith puts the magazine down and approaches Darling.]

BERNITH: Hello

DARLING: Hi

BERNITH: Are you with somebody?

DARLING: I'm sorry?

BERNITH: Who are you here with?

DARLING: I'm alone.

BERNITH: Well, then who are you here to see?

DARLING: I don't know. I've never met him.

BERNITH: Are you visiting?

DARLING: *[Pause]* I hope...I wish...

BERNITH: Oh, you're young, you'll be fine. *[Wanders over toward the men.]* Well, the weather is getting better.

WALLY: Might storm though..

BERNITH: The farmers could use that.

WALLY: Not too much.

RUEBEN: No, you don't want too much.

BERNITH: Well, we're going to get some. Nothing we can do about that..

[Darling walks to the toy box. She absentmindedly starts picking up and touching several things until finally she is holding a cowgirl doll, smoothing its hair and dress. Bernith approaches Darling again.]

BERNITH: That's a pretty dress.

DARLING: *[looks at the doll's dress, then her own.]* My mother...

BERNITH: *[puzzled]* Is it your mother?

DARLING: I don't know. She gave me so much. *[Pause]* She used to make dresses for my babies. They were so delicate . And just look at the pretty hair on this doll.

BERNITH: Is it you?

[Nurse enters.]

NURSE: Darling?

[BERNITH, WALLY, RUEBEN turn to the nurse and say in unison] Yes?

NURSE: [goes toward Darling and touches her shoulder.] Darling?

[Darling puts down the doll]

DARLING: That doll was so easy to take care of. *[Now she looks at the nurse.]* I'm sorry, is it time?

[Nurse leads Darling toward metal door, they exit.]

SONG: verses 3 & 4 of "Is It Time?"
Lyrics by Paul Heckman
Music by Hans Mayer

[verse 3 sung by Mr. Probowski from the back room]
Is it time to lie back down,
Insert the shields and radiate me.
Does this mean we'll be done,

I'll be home by noon?
How do you know that it's time
Don't I have a say in passing?
Can we stop, take a breath, hold each other?

[verse 4 sung by Darling in examining room]
I am sure, if it's time
That the moon will rise and shine
And when it does you and I will keep on loving.
So is it time to draw my blood?
I'll hold still but don't take all day;
I've got things on my mind
And I really cannot stay.

WALLY: There's a storm comin'.

BERNITH: We could use some.

RUEBEN: But not too much.

[NANCY enters, looks around]

NANCY: Where's dad? Did they take him?

RUEBEN: He went in without you. They said it was time.

[Lights dim]

SONG:5 & 6 Is It Time?
Lyrics by Paul Heckman
Music by Hans Mayer

[verse 5 sung by Bernith, Wally, and Rueben]
Is it time? To take a look
At all the causes of this demon;

Find a cure, find a way
To crush its power?
How can it say when it's time
Aren't we stronger than a mutant?
Can we stop, take a breath, hold each other?

[verse 6 sung by Darling]
I am sure, that in time,
While heaven waits for rhyme and reason,
You and I will stop and breathe, and keep on holding.
So is it time? Lead the way.
I will follow but please be kind;
Is this the answer or the end?
And I wonder: is it time?

[Sung by all]
What is it now this time?
I wonder is it time?
What is it now this time?
I wonder is it time?

[Lights up. Nurse enters]

NURSE : Bernith.

[Bernith puts down her magazine, straightens the magazine table, smooths dress. Nurse and Bernith exit through metal door.] [Black out]

Scene 2: Radiation Marking

[Darling is sitting in the examining room. She is looking at a People magazine with a cover that says "The 25 Most Beautiful People". She is wearing a hospital gown and a turban.]

NURSE: *[knocks gently and enters.]* Darling?

DARLING: Yes

NURSE : What are you reading?

DARLING: ... the 25 most beautiful people.

NURSE : Did we make the list?

DARLING: *[Touches her turban.]* No.

NURSE: Well, they're wrong. You know it's all done with computers and airbrushing anyway. They're not perfect. Take my word. I've seen a lot of bodies.

DARLING: I suppose.

NURSE: Well, let's take a look at your glamour shots then. *[X-ray panel projects a computerized image of a body with grids on the neck area.]*

NURSE: This will be your radiation field. We'll use this image to mark you for your first treatment next week.

DARLING: Then will I make the list? *[forced laugh]*

NURSE : A different one maybe – one that matters. Now, lie down and try to relax. I have to mark these coordinates on your skin.

DARLING: *[Lies down on the table.]* How do you mark them?

NURSE: We use a permanent magic marker.

DARLING: Permanent magic...sounds like something I could use right about now.

NURSE : *[Stands over Darling so that audience can no longer see their faces]* Here we go.

[Nurse begins to mark Darling, as she does real photos/video of Darling's neck area appear on the X-ray screen, dark black lines are being drawn on her.]

NURSE: You might want to wear scarves or turtlenecks. These lines go pretty far up your neck and you can't wash them off until we're all done with treatment.

DARLING: What if they start to come off by themselves?

NURSE: Don't worry we'll watch them. We'll see you every day now for the next 4 weeks. If they start to fade we redraw them. I'm almost done here...There that should do it. *[She steps away from Darling.]* You can sit up again for a minute if you'd like.

DARLING: *[Sits up on exam table and looks toward audience.]* Can I have a mirror? I want to see what it's done to me.

NURSE: Are you sure? *[She pulls a hand mirror out of a drawer and hands it to Darling.]*

[Darling looks into the mirror - obscuring her face from the audience - what she is seeing in the mirror is now reflected on one of the X-ray screens.]

DARLING: *[gasps]* Oh, it's so obvious.

NURSE: I know it's kind of a shock at first, but this is the way we do it. It's only for 4 weeks...

DARLING: I know. *[Continues to look in mirror.]* I'm just not sure you got my best angle...don't you want another pose? *[Weak laughter.]*

NURSE: Well, I am going to take another shot. This is one we put up on our patient board. *[She stands off to one side with a digital camera.]*

DARLING: Like this? *[Touches her turban.]*

NURSE: Just like that. We want it to be natural. Just look over here and smile.

DARLING: If I smile it won't be natural.

NURSE: Are you ready? On the count of three...1...2...3 *[Takes shot.]*

DARLING: *[Obviously not relaxed, straightening turban, forced smile.]*

NURSE: That will be great! Do you want to see it? *[Connects camera to computer.]*

DARLING: Thank you...no.

NURSE: Well, I'll email it to you and you can look at it later. *[Works on the computer.]*

DARLING: *[aside]* Yeah, the subject on that email...the 25 most sick...

NURSE: OK, just a few things left to do and then you're done for today. I want to make sure all the equipment we made for you is comfortable.

[She brings out a tray with lead shield, bite bar, arm rests, the tray is labeled 'Darling'.]

NURSE: When you go into the treatment room next week this tray will be there. The technician will put these shields in the machine so that we don't radiate anything we're not supposed to.

DARLING: I always thought we weren't supposed to radiate anything.

NURSE: *[Shows Darling the lead shields and then inserts them into an X-ray machine which she places tightly over Darling's chest.]*

DARLING: They're so thick.

NURSE: That's to protect you.

DARLING: My body was supposed to protect me.

NURSE: Your bottom jaw will be exposed. That could be a problem in the future.

DARLING: A problem?

NURSE: Yes, you will probably lose your bottom teeth. Radiation is pretty hard on your mouth.

DARLING: The doctor never said ...My mouth? My teeth? There are so many things I don't know... but I thought in order to kill the... you know.

NURSE: I know, but you can't worry about that now...first things first. Now these are your arm rests and your bite bar. Let's try them on so you know how to lay.

[She hangs the bite bar from a metal arm above Darling's head and she lays the arm rests next to Darling's head.]

NURSE: You put your arms up into these rests. *[Darling does.]*

Good...just like that...and then the bite bar.

[She lowers the metal arm with the bite bar until it is just above Darling's face]

NURSE: Now, try to reach up and bite on this.

DARLING: *[Dazed]* You said...my teeth

[Darling bites down. Nurse removes Darling's turban and adjusts the level of the bar until she is satisfied.]

NURSE: Is that comfortable?

DARLING: *[says through bite bar]* Comfortable? Look at me!

NURSE: Good job. *[She writes a few things down on a chart.]* We want to make sure you hold perfectly still during treatment...No blurry shots...

[The examining table rises so that Darling faces audience arms at sides, eyes raised, pleading corpse pose. As she does the x-ray panels show a close up of her strained facial expression and then go to the 25 pictures of the patients which includes pictures of Bernith, Wally, Rueben and Mr. Probowski. She puts her hands out beseechingly]

[fade out]

Scene 3: Meet Suddards & Jackie

[Lights come up stage left to reveal a metal scale; a bench with attached table on which blood vials, a rubber tourni- quet and needle drop are visible; a small metal table with a thick patient's file on it, two metal chairs, a bathroom door at the back of the set. There is a full specimen cup in the bathroom]

[Nurse is closing the bathroom door as the scene begins.]

NURSE : Remember the procedure now - wipe, go, collect,

finish, wipe - any questions?

SUDDARDS: *[from behind the wooden door]* Wipe any questions? What...?

NURSE: Just bring it out here when you're finished.

[Nurse moves to the table and begins to sift through the chart.]

NURSE: Mr. Suddards? How are you doing in there?

SUDDARDS: In a minute.

NURSE: Just relax. It's much easier when you relax.

SUDDARDS: It'll be just a minute.

NURSE: Take your time. *[she looks down at her watch.]* Mr. Suddards?

SUDDARDS: Yes.

NURSE: Can I ask you a few questions?

SUDDARDS: I didn't go yet.

NURSE: OK. What's your date of birth?

SUDDARDS: December 6th.

NURSE: Oh, a Sagittarius...stubborn.

SUDDARDS: I'm not not going on purpose.

NURSE: And when did you first notice these symptoms?

SUDDARDS: What?

NURSE: The symptoms...when did you first get sick?

SUDDARDS: I'm not sure. I had this pressure under my right ribs for months...

NURSE: So for awhile now?

SUDDARDS: Ya, but they didn't diagnose it until after the CT scan and now I have to have surgery. *[Pause]* It should all be in my file.

NURSE: I just have to verify things.

SUDDARDS: I know.

NURSE: Do you know who will do your surgery?

SUDDARDS: Don't you? Oh, Dr. Deity.

NURSE: Ohh *[says with admiration]* Dr. Deity...

SUDDARDS: I'm done.

NURSE: Then come out Mr. Suddards and don't forget to flush.

[Sound of toilet flushing, Suddards comes through the bathroom door with a full specimen cup in his hand. He holds it out to the Nurse who sets it on the table.]

NURSE: OK, take your shoes off and now up on the scale.

[Suddards steps out of shoes and onto the scale. Nurse waits for the digital signal from the scale, then jots something down on her clipboard.]

NURSE: You're a pretty big guy.

SUDDARDS: It's hard to fit in....

NURSE: 206 pounds. *[writes it down]* Step over here please. *[Leads Suddards to the bench.]* I need to take some blood. Which arm is better?

SUDDARDS: Uh, what?

NURSE: Which arm?

SUDDARDS: Mine I guess.

[Nurse puts tourniquet on Suddards' right arm and taps the inside of his elbow, looking confused.]

NURSE : You have tiny veins for such a big guy. Are you dehydrated? You know you have to keep drinking. If you drink lots of water before you come in that will help me out, OK? Let's try the other arm.

[She repeats the procedure on Suddards' left arm.]

NURSE: I'm going to try this one, although it's not much better. Now you're going to feel a little poke.
[Suddards winces and looks away from his arm.]

NURSE: I know.

[She fills up 4 vials, then loosens the tourniquet, and puts a gauze wrap on his arm. She writes on each of the vials.]

NURSE: All done.

SUDDARDS: That's my blood? *[stares]* It's so dark.

NURSE: Thank you Mr. Suddards . Now let's get you set up in a room.

[Nurse and Suddards exit to center stage examining room.]

NURSE: *[Takes a hospital gown out of a drawer.]* Take all your clothes off...you can leave your shorts and socks on if you're cold...and put this on. It ties in the back. Dr. Deity's nurse, Jackie, will come in when you're finished.

[Nurse exits with urine specimen and blood vials]

[Suddards goes behind a curtain to change. He emerges in black socks, shorts and a hospital gown. He is not sure where to sit. Goes to the chair and then finally sits on the examining table. He keeps tugging at the gown to make it cover his backside. There is a knock at the stage right door.]

JACKIE: Mr. Suddards, may I come in now?

SUDDARDS: The nurse?

JACKIE: Mr. Suddards, I'm Jackie, Dr. Deity's nurse.

SUDDARDS: Ohh... You're Jackie? a nurse? *[He is obviously surprised that Jackie is male.]*

JACKIE: Yes sir. I'm going to take your blood pressure and ask you a few questions.

[Jackie puts blood pressure cuff on Suddards and pumps it up, lets it release]

JACKIE: Whoa! Are you in there? Let's try it again.

SUDDARDS: Maybe the nurse can help?

JACKIE: *[repeats pumping procedure]* I am a nurse Mr. Suddards. It's just that your pressure is so low...90 over 60. You're pretty calm for all you're facing.

SUDDARDS: *[Looks right at Jackie]* What I'm facing?

JACKIE: Well, sometimes ignorance is bliss, eh?

SUDDARDS: I don't know.

JACKIE: *[Reading and writing in file]* The doctor will tell you everything you need to know. He'll explain all the procedures and risks - then you can make an informed decision.

SUDDARDS: Um, OK. You know, last week I didn't even know where my pancreas was. I guess that's pretty sad.

JACKIE: Not really. Until it flared up there was no reason to pay attention to it. Now, on a scale of 1 to 10 *[shows pain scale picture]* with one being no pain at all and 10 being the worst pain you have ever felt, how would you rate your pain right now?

SUDDARDS: Really it's not so bad - more of a dull ache...a nagging pinch up under my ribs [touches himself]. It's just always there. I've quit wearing my belt. That just seems to aggravate it.

JACKIE: So, on the scale?

SUDDARDS: Do you want a face or a number? I'd say a 3 or 4. *[Jackie points to a face on the scale]*

SUDDARDS: Ya, that guy's about right. It's not too bad...

JACKIE: We don't want you to be a hero. If you're hurting we want to know. We can give you something for the pain if you need it.

SUDDARDS: No, it's OK. It's just gotten sort of familiar.

JACKIE: How's your appetite?

SUDDARDS: Fine.

JACKIE: Bowel movements?

SUDDARDS: *[lools at pain scale again]* Five...

JACKIE: Fine?

SUDDARDS: Yes, fine.

JACKIE: The doctor will be in shortly to discuss your surgery. Now what can I do to make you more comfortable while you wait for him...some water?

[Suddards shakes his head]

JACKIE: A robe?

[Suddards shakes his head.]

JACKIE: A massage

SUDDARDS: What?

JACKIE: Would you like me to give you a massage?

SUDDARDS: *[quickly and emphatically]* No...I mean...No, I'm OK.

[Jackie goes to the desk and writes in the chart. Suddards sits on the examining table. He is obviously nervous, which makes him restless, tugging at his gown and twisting his fingers.]

[Lights down to a lamp on the desk.]

SONG: "That Makes Me A Freak"
Lyrics by Sara M. Slayton
Music by Hans Mayer

Sung by Jackie

The way you look at me,
sir I can tell you're less than pleased.
I'm not what you expected,
my skirt's not short and my hair ain't teased.

But I am a nurse,
and I am a man,
and that makes me a freak.
You question my ability
'cause of my dubious sexuality.

The way I look at it, sir,
I can tell that you need me.
This wasn't what you expected
to get sick and have to lean on me.

But I am a nurse,
and I am a man,
so I want to care for you.

And if that makes me a freak,
I'd rather be odd than to be weak.

[bridge]

I never thought
I could be so strong
to face death every day and not fail.
Is that what a freak is?
A man who wants to relieve pain
and bring a little light to darkened lives?

Well, then I know
I'm a freak. I never feel odd about my job
until someone like you looks at me that way.

I can't change your point of view
but just let me be
and I can care for you.

(bridge)

[Lights up]

JACKIE: You sure there's nothing I can get you?

SUDDARDS: Water.

JACKIE: *[Pours some water.]* Dr. Deity will be here soon. *[He lays his hand on Suddards' shoulder. Suddards draws back from the touch, but Jackie leaves his hand there.]* It's gonna' be alright, sir.

SUDDARDS: *[reaches up and pats Jackie's hand]* Thank you. *[Jackie exits]*

Scene 4: Dr. Deity and Dr. Franco

[There is a slight commotion stage right. Nurse and Jackie are there behind a desk.]

NURSE: *[In an excited whisper]* He's here. He's on the floor. *[Looking around a bit nervously]* Are all the patients prepped?

[Nurse and Jackie straighten things around them and themselves. Music builds as Dr. Deity, Dr. Franco, and 2 interns enter from the right through an elevator type door.]

[choreography = Dr. Franco steps off elevator ahead of Dr. Deity. He holds a wet umbrella which he folds up and shakes out 'like holy water' in front of Dr. Deity. Dr. Deity has a coat draped over his shoulders, which an intern whisks away while the nurse drapes a lab coat in its place.. The interns and Dr. Franco circle around Deity, parting the way for him, taking notes, nodding, affirming - all 'in time' to his movements. Dr. Deity stops at the nurses' station — nurse straightens things and fusses. Dr. Deity puts out his hand and Jackie places a clipboard in it and then joins the entourage. They look at charts, Deity whispers to Jackie and Dr. Franco, they write up orders and all move on]

Song: Dr. Deity
Lyrics by Paul Heckman
Music by Hans Mayer

[verse 1 sung by Dr. Franco]
Folks, clear the way,
Step aside for the man
who can work miracles, and he has.
Show some respect
for the man in the suit
who gives cancer the boot, let him pass.
It's a miracle
and there ain't no doubt
We're all here to serve
And on call to shout:

[refrain sung by all]
Doctor D! Doctor D! Doctor De - i -ety
Hand him your X-rays
and count on your next days
'cause he is the one
count on him son
to get the job done.

[verse 2 sung by interns]
Soon, with heavenly grace
Like a hand from above
He pulls on a glove
And he grins.
Shine – glorious light
Steal the dark from the night
Everything is all right – let's begin
Standing tall and bold
Like the man upstairs
You have got to know
He's the one who spares.

[refrain sung by all]

[verse 3 spoken by Dr. Deity]
What we got here is an evil beast
And when I look in its face
My wrath is unleashed
'cause that's how I operate.
And if that evil has spread
I just gather my will
And nod my sweet head
'cause that's how I operate.

[sung by interns]
Ask the nurses now,
They will always say
'cause his heart is pure
he has saved the day.

[refrain sung by all]

[Dr. Franco knocks on Suddards' examining room door.]

DR. FRANCO: Mr. Suddards are you ready?

SUDDARDS: *[Quickly sits down.]* For?

[Dr. Deity and entourage enter the examining room, Dr. Franco is always at his right hand. Suddards draws his gown tighter around him.]

DR. DEITY: Hello, Mr. Suddards. *[Holds out his hand.]* I'm Dr. Deity. I'll be performing your surgery.

SUDDARDS: *[Takes his hand.]*

DR. DEITY: Good. This is my resident, Dr. Fanco. He will assist me in the operating room. And these are interns working with me. They will be observing your exam today. And you've met my nurse, Jackie?.

SUDDARDS: Yes. So many of you...*[pulls gown tighter]*

DR. FRANCO: Now, do you know why you're here today Mr. Suddards?

SUDDARDS: Something is wrong...Oh, I mean to discuss an operation...my operation.

 DR. FRANCO: That's right. It's called a Whipple procedure. Let me show you how it works, *[He takes out a pen and clipboard.. What he draws is projected on the x-ray screens]* This is your pancreas. It's located between your stomach and your small intestine. You have a 30 millimeter tumor, about the size of a grape, in the head of your pancreas - about here- that is malignant and has to be removed. Now in order to do that we have to remove part of your stomach, your gall bladder, part of your bile duct and your duodenum. Do you understand?

SUDDARDS: Understand? Uh, I guess...pancreas, gall, bile... no. Maybe I don't...

DR. FRANCO: That's where the doctor comes in. The doctor is in the details.

[Dr. Deity leans over and makes a very small change to Dr. Franco's drawing]

DR. FRANCO: Oh, yes. *[Interns give a 'knowing' look]*

SUDDARDS: Looks like plumbing. Have to reroute a lot of pipes.

DR. DEITY: *[terse smile]* It's more than plumbing.

DR. FRANCO: Yes. It should take about 10 hours.

SUDDARDS: So long... *[Jackie comes over to Suddards' bedside and stands by him]*

DR. FRANCO: As you said, a lot of connections to repair. While we're in there we'll also remove and biopsy about 15 of your surrounding lymph nodes just to make sure this thing hasn't metastasized - spread. Then we close you up and it's all over for awhile.

SUDDARDS: Awhile?

DR. DEITY: Then you rest. Probably a 9 or 10 day stay at the hospital. Once we know you're healing and all your systems are working again you can go home. We'll let you recuperate for about 10 days and then we'll see you after that. Any questions?

SUDDARDS: So much to remember. *[Pause]* Will this... will this scare me?

DR. FRANCO: You mean a scar? Yes. We have to start the cut

about here *[touches Suddards who reacts with a wince]* and continue all the way across to the other side *[draws finger all across Suddards' stomach]* It's the only way.

SUDDARDS: *[now visibly nervous/shaken]* What about problems?

DR. FRANCO: Complications? Well, it's more than plumbing. Anytime we cut into major organs like this there is a possibility of problems. In this situation it could be excessive bleeding, infection, or the onset of post- operative diabetes.

DR. DEITY: *[Deity looks right into Suddards' face]* Mr. Suddards you have to trust me to do this right. It's what I've trained for all my life and I'm damned good at it.

SUDDARDS: Are there...ummm...I mean, odds?

DR. FRANCO: 70% of people come through the surgery without major complications. *[Jackie puts his hand on Suddards' shoulder, Suddards does not react]*

DR. DEITY: My personal rate is closer to 80%.

SUDDARDS: And the cancer? How many...?

DR. FRANCO: You want to know? *[Suddards nods]* Well...

DR. DEITY: About 2 in 5 make it past the first 5 years.

[Interns and Suddards gasp aloud, Dr. Franco looks away, Suddards reaches up and touches Jackie's hand]

SUDDARDS: Not so good...

DR. DEITY: Will you let me help you Mr. Suddards?

SUDDARDS: Help? Oh yes, yes.

DR. DEITY: Good. I can do this for you a week from tomorrow.

SUDDARDS: Already?

DR. DEITY: Waiting serves no real purpose.

SUDDARDS: Oh, no real purpose...

DR. DEITY: OK then, Jackie will get everything set up with you. Until next week?

[Deity & Suddards shake hands, Dr. Franco does the same; they and the interns exit]

JACKIE: I'll give you a few minutes to get dressed. Then I'll come back in and tell you all about getting prepared for the surgery.

[Jackie exits, leaving Suddards sitting alone on the examining table. Stage darkens to a single spot on him as he gets up and goes to the drawings on the x-ray screens. He traces a few lines with his finger and begins to sway as the music begins]

Song: Tropical Cancer
Lyrics by Paul D. Heckman
Music by Hans Mayer

[Sung softly by Suddards]
On Col O Gee, On Col O Gee
They look/ for signs/ inside of me.
On Col O Gee, On Col O Gee,
Oh what/ size fruit's/ inside of me?

Bio Op See, Bio Op See,
Oh what/ size fruit's/ inside of me?
Bio Op See, Bio Op See,
They look/ for signs/ inside of me.

They are so wise, to name the size –
A lemon, a lime, a grape this time?
They are astute, their point is moot -
Wow!/ You've got/ a ripe grapefruit!

An orange, a cherry, a huckleberry,
What's on/ that tree/ inside of me?
A mango, pineapple, I sound like Snapple,
Oh ya/ it's Straw/ berry/ Kiwi

On Col O Gee, Bio Op See,
A citrus fruit/ menagerie.
Bio Op See, On Col O Gee,
This fruit/ is not/ so good for me.

Bio Op See, On Col O Gee,
This fruit/ is not/so good for me.
On Col O Gee, Bio Op See,
Harvest/ this mess/ inside of me.

[After the song Suddards lies down on the bed, still dim lit
stage. Jackie enters in scrubs, covers Suddards up, attaches
breathing tubes, turns bed around. Dr. Deity and Dr. Franco &
interns enter wearing scrubs, with gloves raised in the air. They
reprise the Dr. Deity song [sung very softly by all, as Deity
performs surgery, with spot light on him entire time. Dr.
Deity's spoken verse is intense and determined. Everyone
dressed in scrubs, masks, moving around the body, handing
things to Dr. Deity. Several monitoring machines are working.]

Scene 5: Mr. Probowski's Daughter

(Spot on Mr. Probowski sitting in a wheelchair at the front of the stage. He is napping, head bowed. He is completely bald and a deep red scar cuts across his scalp. His breathing is shallow and somewhat erratic.)

(Nancy enters quietly. She is wearing a cap and coat]

NANCY: Dad? *[pause]* Dad? *[She gently nudges his shoulder.]*

MR. PROBOWSKI: What? *[Slowly comes to]* Time?

NANCY: Just about. I brought this blanket. It's a bit chilly outside. *[She tucks the blanket around him]*

MR. PROBOWSKI: ...time is it?

NANCY: It's almost time.

MR. PROBOWSKI: *[Looks down at and touches blanket.]* For bed?

NANCY: No, no, dad. I just thought you'd want this blanket when we go outside. We're going for your treatment in just a few minutes. Do you remember?

MR. PROBOWSKI: Yes, getting the treatment.

NANCY: You'll get to see all your nice friends at the clinic.

MR. PROBOWSKI: They're patients.

NANCY: Well, they're a nice bunch anyway, and I know you like talking to them.

MR. PROBOWSKI: So much in common. We're all falling apart

in one room together. Now that's what I call close.

NANCY: Well, I like them and I've gotten to know them pretty well. Heck, I see them every day. That's more than I see my own friends.

MR. PROBOWSKI: I know...I know...You don't have much of a life these days either, taking care of me all the time. Who'd have thought my last group of friends would be such a bunch of sick bastards.

NANCY: Dad! I want to take care of you, you know that. Don't you worry about me.

MR. PROBOWSKI: Maybe we can't help it.

NANCY: Well, now it's time to let me concentrate on you for awhile...it's only fair.

MR. PROBOWSKI: Remember we went to Toronto for the conference? How old were you? 10? That was a great time. You kept a silly little journal on the trip. I still have it in my desk and you sang and your mother....your mother was so beautiful....

NANCY: It was a great trip Dad...one of my favorites. I still have the snow globe we bought there, and I miss mom, too. But maybe I'm glad she's not here right now...

MR. PROBOWSKI: She was too beautiful for this.

NANCY: So, all ready to go? *[Approaches Probowski and gives him a kiss on the head.]* It's cold out there today. Oh, speaking of the cold, I brought you a present. *[Holds out a wrapped box]*

MR. PROBOWSKI: *[Looks at her and the present]* For me? getting it about half unwrapped.]*

NANCY: Here dad, let me help you with that. *[She finishes pulling off the paper and ribbon.]*

MR. PROBOWSKI: What the...?

NANCY: A hat dad. And not just any hat *[She holds up the hat. It is a black wool captain's cap with a long braid of red hair attached to the back of it.]* It's one of a kind. A genuine Probowski! Just like you!

MR. PROBOWSKI: *[Holds the hat and looks at it. Finally he touches the long braid and looks at Nancy.]*

NANCY: *[Takes off her cap to reveal short red hair.]* That's right dad, it's my hair. Our hair. You gave it to me, I'm giving it back to you.

MR. PROBOWSKI: Our hair...oh...

NANCY: Here, let's put it on. *[She puts the cap on his head.]* Oh, dad you look 20 years younger!

MR. PROBOWSKI: Great! Who wants to look like a 72 year old man? Thank you honey. Thank you.

NANCY: Are you ready dad? It's almost time.

MR. PROBOWSKI: Ya time.

NANCY: Here we go. *[She wheels him off]*

Scene 6: Radiation Waiting Room

[Lights up on the radiation waiting room set as before, but a different day. The 4 people are seated in the exact same seats. Darling enters, she is now wearing a wig. Bernith, Wally,

Mr. Probowski, Rueben all look up and their expressions soften. Mr. Probowski is in his wheel chair, wearing his cap and looking more ill.]

BERNITH: Good morning Darling. Don't you look pretty?

DARLING: *[Touches her wig.]* Do you like it? I mean, does it look natural?

BERNITH: Oh, yes. It's very attractive on you. No one would ever know.

DARLING: Except for us of course. *[Darling touches Bernith's hand.]*

BERNITH: My sister read that when your hair comes back after chemo it's always different...redder and curlier, too.

DARLING: I could handle that. Then I'd look like Mr. Probowski's beautiful daughter. *[She approaches Mr. Probowski and "pets" his ponytail]* Or maybe like you...look at this beautiful braid. I love how it's tied.

MR. PROBOWSKI: *[weakly]* I go on trial today.

DARLING: What?

MR. PROBOWSKI: On trial.

BERNITH: They're moving him onto trial drugs today. Nothing else is working. Those drugs are supposed to be pretty good...in those really extreme cases...I mean...

MR. PROBOWSKI: *[slowly & weakly]* I'm in the extreme – Yeah!.

BERNITH: *[flustered and embarrassed]* Oh...I didn't really mean anything...oh...

DARLING: Bernith, now is not the time.

[Nurse enters]

NURSE: Mr. Probowski?

MR. PROBOWSKI: *[Looks back at others.]* I know.

[Nurse and Mr. Probowski exit through metal door.]

BERNITH: *[Goes over to sit by Darling and takes her hand.]* Tell me about your week. Have you been eating? 'Cause you gotta eat to keep your strength up. All the reports say that you've gotta eat to keep your strength up. What are you eating?

DARLING: I had some fruit. Some Clementine oranges. They were so good.

BERNITH: Juicy...good...easy to peel.

WALLY: I'm allergic to oranges.

RUEBEN: What difference does that make now?

BERNITH: Well, you gotta' eat to keep your strength up. You gotta' be strong. *[Pause]* I'll bring cookies.

WALLY: Don't put any oranges in them.

RUEBEN: What difference does it make?

DARLING: That would be wonderful, Bernith.

[Darling wanders over to the jigsaw puzzle on the table. She starts picking up pieces and trying to fit them in.]

VOLUNTEER: *[Enters, waters the plant, sweeps up the dead leaves, throws them in a wastebasket near the puzzle table.]* Do you like puzzles?

DARLING: Some. I don't like things I can't solve, though.

VOLUNTEER: Well, I'll just warn you, there may be some pieces missing.

DARLING: Welcome to my world...*[distant]*

[Nurse enters]

NURSE: Darling?

[Darling waves to Bernith and exits with nurse through metal door.]

BERNITH: *[Picks up a magazine and looks at the cover]* Pretty girl...so young...

WALLY: She looks like my wife years ago.

BERNITH: Why so young?

RUEBEN: Why anybody?

WALLY: *[pause]* I get a rash from strawberries, too.

BERNITH: *[picks up another magazine and looks at cover]* This one looks so healthy. She looks like Darling.

WALLY: No peanuts either.

RUEBEN: Ya, that girl's got the right name. She's the darling of this crowd.

BERNITH: So pretty.

(Instrumental intro to "Darling of the Waiting Room" begins quietly. Bernith begins to softly hum and gently sway as she rearranges the magazine table.]

BERNITH: And so young.

[Rueben stands, starts to hum harmony and sidles over to Bernith.]

RUEBEN: Be careful of your hip now.

WALLY: I hate waiting.

BERNITH: Waiting is hard but we have all this room.

[Lights dim]

Song: The Darling of the Waiting Room
Lyrics by Sara M. Slayton
Music by Hans Mayer

(Bernith & Rueben sway as they sing the refrain and 1st verse)
Boop, Bop, Boop, Bop
Boop, Bop, Boop, Bop
Boop, Bop, Boop, Bop

Here we are
in the waiting room
every day - in limbo land.
This is the place
where people come
to wait their lives away.
It's a junction,
where the patients meet
and with forced smiles
we try to stay up beat.

(Bernith & Rueben sing and dance)
Boop, Bop, Boop, Bop
Boop, Bop, Boop, Bop
Boop, Bop, Boop, Bop
Boop, Bop, Boop, Bop

(Wally sings)
There is a girl
who comes each day
She's so sweet - we wait for her.
She's so young
we can believe
that everything's OK.
She's the darling
of the waiting room.
Such a darling,
our poster girl.

(Wally dances and sings refrain with Bernith)

(All sing)
Here we are
in the waiting room
every day - in limbo land.
This is the place
she brings us hope,
She's got to be OK.

(bridge)

(All sing & dance)
She smiles at me
and takes my hand.
How can it be?
I don't understand.

She shouldn't be here
where people come
to wait their lives away.
She's the darling
of the waiting room.
Such a darling,
our poster girl.

(All sing refrain& dance)

End of Act One

Act Two:

Scene 1: Coffee Shop

[Stage left. A typical coffee shop...small tables, flowers, counter, artwork]

[Cyan, Mary Catherine are seated at a table, drinking coffee. Mary Catherine is working on a lap top computer open in front of her.]

MARY CATHERINE: Almost done...*[She hits a few more keys and then closes the computer.]* Sorry about that.

CYAN: Oh, I don't mind. I'm in no hurry

MARY CATHERINE: I thought you had somewhere to go.

CYAN: Just errands...but I thought I might stop to see Darling.

MARY CATHERINE: I should do that one of these days. I keep meaning to call and schedule a time, but I never get to it.

CYAN: Do you think we have to schedule our visits? I was hoping I could just stop by....if I didn't stay too long...

MARY CATHERINE: I'm sure that's fine. I just have so much on my plate I can hardly squeeze extra things in. You know how it is, if it's not on my planner I don't do it. How did we ever get so busy?

CYAN: I'm not sure. It can't be good for any of us.   Maybe that's what's wrong with Darling. She just got going too fast. Maybe this will slow her down.

MARY CATHERINE: Well, it's done that!

CYAN: I didn't mean anything by that. I just meant all this rushing around... it's just not good...for any of us. Do you think I should take her something? Maybe a good book or some flowers?

MARY CATHERINE: She loves her garden.

CYAN: Yes, some spring bulbs. That should cheer her up. I'll stop at Crane's Nursery on the way over and pick some up.

MARY CATHERINE: I haven't been there in ages. They always have such nice things. She'll like that.

CYAN: Daffodils would be nice. A sunny color.

MARY CATHERINE: *[Looks around for waitress.]* Do you want something? I'm a bit hungry. You, know the last time I saw Darling she was awfully thin. I suppose that can't be helped. I offered to lend her some of mine *[She pats her belly, both laugh.]*

[Waitress comes to table]

MARY CATHERINE: I'll take one of those chocolate swirl biscottis.

WAITRESSS: They're two for the price of one today.

MARY CATHERINE: Cyan?

CYAN: Why not? I deserve it. *[laughter]*

MARY CATHERINE: Better make it two then, thanks. *[Pause]* Do you think she's eating anything these days?

CYAN: I don't know. She used to love bread. You know, hard, crusty, European style stuff. The heavier the better.

MARY CATHERINE: I know! And she never gained a pound, that little shit. I just look at those loaves and I swell up. Well, I guess this is one time that I'm glad I'm not skinny...I mean, you know...

CYAN: She has so little to fight with.

[Enter Mona. She bustles in with several parcels which she sets in the empty chair.]

MONA: I'm so sorry. I started out on time, but...

MARY CATHERINE: We never expect you on time you know.

MONA: That's not fair. I just get so busy.

CYAN: So distracted you mean. [laughter]

MONA: It's like time disappears. I think I have all the time in the world and then I look at the clock and it has all just slipped away.

MARY CATHERINE: You try to do too much at once. You always figure you can do things in half the time it really takes. You have to be more realistic.

MONA: Well, if that means being hooked up all the time [points at the computer] then no thanks. I heard the other day you can get brain cancer from being on the cell phone all the time.

CYAN: I'm planning on stopping by to see Darling today.

MONA: Really? I didn't say that brain cancer thing about her you know. You're braver than I am. I would love to talk to her but I just can't be around sick people. It makes me queasy. How awful is that? Do you think I'm an awful person?

MARY CATHERINE: It's just honest. You wouldn't do her any good if you were freaking out. She needs stable people around her, not nervous wrecks.

MONA: I wouldn't do her any good.

CYAN: But she needs her friends. Especially now – she needs us.

MONA: Maybe she just needs her rest. I know when I'm sick I just need to be alone.

MARY CATHERINE: Not me. I want someone to fuss over me and pamper me...a lot!

MONA: See? That's just it. How can we know what she wants or needs? It's better not to intrude. Besides if she looks sick...like no hair...I won't know where to look.
[there is a lull in the conversation]

MARY CATHERINE: I was just saying that the last time I saw her she was so thin.

MONA: Well, I can do that! I can make her some food. Then I could bring it here and one of you could take it to her. I can do that. What do you think she'd like?

CYAN: That's just it, we don't know. I guess I could ask her today. Maybe she'll have some ideas and then I can call you later.

MONA: That's what I can do.

MARY CATHERINE: I think that's for the best.

CYAN: I better go if I'm going to get everything done and still have time to stop at Darling's. Here's for the coffee.
[Puts down some bills.]

MONA: But I just got here...sorry I was so late. *[Looks to Cyan]* Be sure to call me later.

MARY CATHERINE: That's too much...and what about the biscotti?

CYAN: *[as she leaves]* Share them with Mona. She could use the calories and the rest. *[laughter]*

MARY CATHERINE: Bye. Tell her hello.

MONA: For me, too.

[Cyan exits.]

[Lights lower to a spot on Mary Catherine as she opens up her computer and begins typing. As she does she sings the first verse of "If You Need Anything, Just Ask"]

SONG: If You Need Anything, Just Ask
Lyrics by Sara M. Slayton
Music by Hans Mayer

(Sung by Mary Catherine)
Oh, I just heard that you were sick and I
meant to call for so long.
I don't know why I didn't but I've been
so busy every day.
You know I think of you,
but it makes me feel so blue,
so let me say,
"It will turn out fine. It will turn out fine. It will turn out fine.
If you need anything, just ask
It will turn out fine. It will turn out fine, It will turn out fine."

(bridge)

[The spot shifts to Mona handing a casserole to Cyan.]

(Mona, sings the second verse)
Have you seen her lately? I just
can't go there by myself.
Sick people scare me half to death and I
never know what to say.
If she looks in my eyes
I will just start to cry,
so let me say,
"Send her my greetings. Send her my greetings. Send her my
greetings.
If she needs anything, just ask.
Send her my greetings. Send her my greetings. Send her my
greetings."
(bridge)

*[The spot shifts to Cyan arriving at a door which Darling
answers. She hands her the casserole and daffodils}*

Cyan sings the third verse]
How good to see you, you look great for all
that you've been through lately.
I'm rather curious to see your scar but
I don't know just how to ask.
And when I look at you
I feel so guilty,
so let me say,
"You will recover. You will recover. You will recover.
If you need anything, just ask.
You will recover. You will recover. You will recover."

(bridge)

*[Cyan leaves and Darling leans up against the door with a
casserole and flowers in her hands. She sings the rest of the
song]*

(Darling sings)
I know you all mean well and I thank you
for your thoughts and prayers,
and for the casseroles and books and cards.
I appreciate them all.
But if you want to know
what I could use right now
just let me say,
"I want to grow old. I want to grow old. I want to grow old.
I'm asking for a cure.
I want to grow old. I want to grow old. I want to grow old."

 (bridge)

"I want to grow old. I want to grow old. I want to grow old.
I'm asking for a cure.
I want to grow old. I want to grow old. I want to grow old."

Scene 2: Suddards' Post Op

*(Suddards is in the examining room. He has visibly lost
weight. He is wearing a hospital gown, sitting on the
exam table, slumped and obviously weaker]*

[Knock at the door]

JACKIE: Mr. Suddards may I come in now?

SUDDARDS: Nurse? Yes.

JACKIE: *[enters and shakes Suddards' hand]* Good to see
you again, sir. *[sits down and opens file]* So how have you
been doing since surgery?

SUDDARDS: OK. Mama used to call me her big boy.

JACKIE: Any blood in your urine or stool?

SUDDARDS: No.

JACKIE: *[he writes in the file as he talks]* Regular bowel movements?

SUDDARDS: Wait. What? Regular bowels...yes.

JACKIE: *[sets down file and approaches Suddards]* May I see your incision please?

[Suddards lifts his gown to reveal a deep red scar all across the front of his body. He is obviously modest and somewhat uncomfortable with this.]

JACKIE: *[Touches the scar.]* Any pain here?

SUDDARDS: I can't feel anything...it's all numb. Am I supposed to feel something?

JACKIE: Not really. Some of the nerves were severed and others...well, it just takes time.

SUDDARDS: Everything does, I guess.

JACKIE: *[Looks away from Suddards face.]* Now let's take your vitals. Up on the scale please, *[weighs him and notes it in the file]* You've lost a bit. *[Jackie takes Suddards' wrist and counts pulse silently]* Your pulse is fine. *[Jackie puts on blood pressure cuff and pumps it up]* 102 over 70, still pretty low.

SUDDARDS: That's good right?

JACKIE: Absolutely. Your system is still pretty calm despite everything you've been through.

SUDDARDS: Don't feel very calm...

JACKIE: Well, your surgery went very well. I think you have every reason to be calm. So you just stay that way and the doctor will be in shortly. Is there anything you need?

SUDDARDS: Maybe a robe.

JACKIE: Sure. *[He gets a robe out of a drawer]* Here you go.

SUDDARDS: Thank you Jackie.

[Jackie exits. Suddards stands up slowly, holding his belly. He puts on the robe, it obviously hurts him to twist/turn. He sits back down and absentmindedly rubs his belly.]

[Knock at the door]

DR. DEITY: Mr. Suddards? *[He enters with Dr. Franco, the intern and Jackie. Dr. Deity shakes Suddards' hand]* You remember my resident, Dr. Franco? *[They shake hands]* And my interns? *[they nod at one another]*

SUDDARDS: Yes.

DR. DIETY: Well, you look pretty good. Now, how long ago was that surgery? *[He looks to Dr. Franco]*

SUDDARDS: Five...six...

DR. FRANCO: *[Looking in Suddards' file]* Six weeks ago this Friday. We gave him a little extra time at home to heal.

DR. DEITY: So, how have you been feeling since then?

SUDDARDS: Pretty tired at first...

DR. FRANCO: It was a major surgery Mr. Suddards. You were in the operating room for over 9 hours. It takes a while to come back from that.

SUDDARDS: Coming back?

DR. FRANCO: *[Sits down with chart]* Well, let's see now. All your blood work looks pretty good at this stage of the game. Some of your levels are a bit elevated, but that's to be expected. The best news is that the tumor marker test is within the normal range.

SUDDARDS: *[Looks baffled.]* Normal..?

DR. FRANCO: That means we think we got all the cancer with surgery. Lucky for you, you had pain. Usually patients don't feel anything until it's too late. Let me show you the scans. *[Dr. Franco puts them up on the projection x-ray screens.]* This was your abdominal scan prior to surgery. See this? That was the tumor. We took it out along with 15 lymph nodes so that now it looks like this *[Points to another scan.]* This is your scan from last week.

SUDDARDS: Normal...

DR. DEITY: It's what I do. Now let's take a look at you. *[Puts stethoscope to Suddards' back and chest and does the breathing thing.]* Could you lie down please?

JACKIE: *[Steps up and takes Suddards' arm to help him lie down.]*

DR. DEITY: *[Pulls up Suddards' gown to reveal his underwear and belly. Suddards is obviously embarrassed by everyone looking at him and turns his head away from them. Dr. Deity runs his fingers along Suddards' scar.]* This looks really good Mr. Suddards. Any oozing or unusual pain along the incision?

SUDDARDS: Unusual? What's...no.

DR. DEITY: Any belly aches?

SUDDARDS: No.

DR. DEITY: Diarrhea or constipation?

SUDDARDS: Uh, constipation, a little.

DR. DEITY: Are you still taking pain medication?

SUDDARDS: Sometimes at night...yes.

DR. DIETY: That's probably the culprit then. *[Looks at Dr. Franco]* Write up a prescription for Senna. It's a natural laxative. It should help. How much weight have you lost since surgery?

SUDDARDS: I don't know. Got new holes in my belt. *[Feeble smile.]*

DR. DIETY: *[Looking in file.]* 206 to 163...that's umm...43 pounds. That's in the normal range. You can figure on a permanent weight loss of about 25%. How's your appetite?

SUDDARDS: I get hungry but...I can't eat much.

DR. DIETY: You'll probably eat less, but more often. We had to reduce the size of your stomach and reroute your intestine. You've got all new plumbing down there *[smile]*. You can sit up. *[Jackie helps Suddards sit up]* Now, let's talk about your treatment.

SUDDARDS: But you said you got everything with surgery.

DR. DIETY: Yes, as far as we can tell things look good.

SUDDARDS: But... the tumor marker... test?

DR. DIETY: Even that can only detect things after a certain amount of activity has already occurred. In fact you'd have to have nearly a million abnormal cells for them to show up on that. I don't think you want to risk iit

SUDDARDS: Never did...

DR. FRANCO: We are usually aggressive with this thing. It has a way of hiding.

DR. DEITY: Figure on at least 8 courses of chemo and a month of radiation. [Suddards reacts with a wince.] Jackie will go through all the particulars with you and set up the appointments. I'll want to see you again about halfway through your chemo. We'll do another belly scan then too. [Stands to leave.] OK then Mr. Suddards? We're all set? [Holds out his hand.]

SUDDARDS: [Shakes Dr. Deity's hand and Dr. Franco's hand.] Halfway...normal...OK

[Dr. Deity, Dr. Franco and intern leave - Jackie is last]

JACKIE: [turns to Suddards] Are you alright Mr. Suddards?

SUDDARDS: Alright...normal...OK

JACKIE: I'll give you a few minutes to get dressed and then I'll be back to set up those chemo appointments. [exits]

Scene 3: Boomer's Questions

[Stage right - The radiation waiting room.]

[Wally and Rueben are seated in their usual places. Mr.

Probowski's wheelchair is obviously vacant and avoided as other characters walk near it.]

[Darling's chair is also empty]

[Volunteer enters, waters plant and sweeps up the fallen leaves, goes to aquarium to feed the fish, notices one is dead, gets net and scoops it out, wraps it up in Kleenex and carries it away.]

[Bernith gets up and puts cookies out on the table]

[Center stage - dimly lit. Suddards sits in a wheel chair with IV pole next to him]

BERNITH: I brought cookies.

WALLY: Darling's all done. Her last treatment was Wednesday.

BERNITH: I know, but I thought you boys would miss it if I didn't bring a treat. Anyway we could all use a few extra calories. Gotta' keep our strength up...all the books say...

RUEBEN: We know...we know.

BERNITH: Oatmeal, but no raisins. I know you don't like raisins.

WALLY: Or nuts.

BERNITH: No nuts either. They're pretty plain, but they're healthy - good for you, you know.

RUEBEN: Good for me. Bad for me. Up, down, six of one....

[Bernith goes to pour some coffee.]

[A new character (Boomer) enters. He is wearing a continuous drip chemo cassette and a Rock & Roll T-shirt. You can see the intravenous line running into his elbow. He has long hair/ ponytail, an earring and baggy jeans]

[Center stage - Jackie hooks Suddards up to intravenous chemo bag]

BERNITH: Oh, hello.

BOOMER: Hi.

BERNITH: Are you visiting?

BOOMER: No.

BERNITH: *[Looks toward Wally and Rueben]* Well, are you here to see...?

BOOMER: The doctor.

BERNITH: Oh...*[recognition that he is a patient]* Oh...

BOOMER: First day of radiation.

BERNITH: *[Leads him to what used to be Darling's chair]* Well, you sit down right here. That's where all the newcomers sit. It's good luck.

BOOMER: Good luck? I'll remember that.

RUEBEN: Ya, people go home from that chair.

BERNITH: I made oatmeal cookies. I'll get you one. *[She goes to the table, gets a cookie and napkin and returns to Boomer]*

BOOMER: I'd love to, really, but I can't. Sorry. I can't seem to eat anything hard..*[points to his mouth]* my mouth.

BERNITH: I'm sorry. I eat OK, I just can't seem to stay awake...taking naps all day, like a baby.

RUEBEN: He's on chemo. That's why he gets mouth sores. Can't you see?

BERNITH: *[Looks at Boomer's arm and cassette]* Oh...

RUEBEN: I had mouth sores, too. Try popsicles.

BOOMER: I heard that. But they go away?

WALLY: The popsicles?

RUEBEN: Sort of. Mostly you just get used to it. I lost 22 pounds during chemo. Kind of lost my interest in food. Tasted like metal.

BOOMER: That's the truth.

BERNITH: Oh, that's the worst. I'm glad I didn't have to do that - chemo, I mean. People say it's worse than the cancer...all that pain and vomiting... I couldn't stand it. *[She takes a bite of a cookie]*

[There is an awkward lull]

[On center stage Jackie is wiping Suddard's forehead with a towel. Suddenly Suddards starts retching, takes towel to mouth and Suddards throws up.]

BOOMER: Actually my chemo hasn't been too bad so far. This little pump puts it in one drop at a time...all day and night. S'posed to make it a little easier.

RUEBEN: *[Gets up and goes to look at Boomer's chemo cassette set up]* That's a real improvement alright. I got my chemo once every three weeks - all the drugs at once. Took them 3 hours to push them all through my system. Go in on Thursdays, get shot full of chemo and spend the next 24 hours sleeping in the bathtub...so I'd be near the toilet. Sometimes I threw up for 36 hours straight.

[Suddards wretches and vomits again center stage]

BOOMER: Man!

WALLY: It's poison you know.

RUEBEN: Ya, well your body knows that for sure. It gets rid of it anyway it can - runny nose, watery eyes - whatever it takes. Even my sweat smelled funny. Like metal.

BOOMER: Well, I'm sure glad for this little gizmo then. I haven't had any of that - except for some bouts of nausea and now these mouth sores.

RUEBEN: Try popsicles.

WALLY: Or ice chips – they always have them here.

BERNITH: Maybe I'll make some lemon bars, they're soft. *[Looks at Wally]* Can you eat lemon?

WALLY: I like lemon pudding. I used to like Tapioca, but I haven't had that for years.

BERNITH: Or maybe angel food cake. That's soft too...

[They all sit in silence for a bit]

BOOMER: I read about, you know...but what's the radiation like?

RUEBEN: Not as bad as chemo. It doesn't make you sick.

BERNITH: Just sleepy.

BOOMER: But this whole radiation thing is pretty scary. I mean, I grew up in the 60s...you know, the Cold War and all the H-bomb stuff. I can remember having civil defense drills in school. In case of an attack we were supposed to crawl under the pews in the church and put our hands over our heads. We would have been an orderly group of charred biscuits if anything had ever happened.

ALL: *[polite laughter]*

BOOMER: But I mean it. We were taught to be afraid of radiation...not to go near it. Now I'm gonna lie down in some room and let them shoot it at me. How can this be helping? Wasn't one of the scares of atomic survival that we'd all come down with cancer?

WALLY: But it's all we got...we have to trust them...

RUEBEN: I don't know. They all run out of the room before they turn on the machine...they don't want to be near it.

WALLY: Better not to think about it too much. It upsets your stomach.

[On center stage, Suddards has one last wretch and then Jackie wheels him off]

BOOMER: *[Boomer gets up and walks over to the aquarium,*

brushes his hand over the glass, looks at the fish]
I remember when all it took was a baby aspirin.

SONG:Boomer's Got A Question
Lyrics by Paul D. Heckman
Music by Hans Mayer

Mommy said it's dangerous
Daddy said it too,
But the doctors and nurses
Assure me the purpose
Is only to help pull me through.
When I ask if it's safe now
Well, they smile and they wink
As if to say, "in this place, man,
It's better not to think."

I'm just worried and wonderin' how bad can turn out good
Does radiation somehow know
To do the things we say we know it should
With its luminescent glow?

Momma says it's painless
Daddy nods his head,
And the doctors and nurses
Assure me the curse is
Being sick means at least I'm not dead.
When I ask them what has changed,
Why is nuking me O.K.?
I see their faces look ashamed
Before they look away.

I'm just worried and wonderin' how you came to decide
Does radiation really find
The senseless, scary growth I have inside
How can evil be so kind?

So here I am just asking,
Not to contradict;
Can the doctors and nurses
Assure me the worst is
The best they can do for the sick?

Yes, I still have a question
As they place the shield of lead
Can something bring me back to life
That's meant to make us dead?

I'm just worried and wonderin' about what I used to hear
Can radiation be all right?
Can something we all once claimed to fear
Be cast in such a light?

Scene 4: Suddards' Hospice

[Transform stage left into a living room. Window frames are placed alongside door at back of set, a hospital bed, soft chair, small throw rug, lamp, end table, plant are added. Jackie is sitting in the chair, Suddards is lying on the bed asleep, slowly coming to.]

JACKIE: Mr. Suddards? *[No answer.]* Mr. Suddards are you waking up?

SUDDARDS: Up.

JACKIE: Good, then let's change your clothes. *[Goes over to the bed and begins to get Suddards sitting upright.]*

SUDDARDS: Why?

JACKIE: Well, you've been sleeping in them all night. Fresh pajamas will feel better.

SUDDARDS: *(Looks down at himself)* Oh.

[Jackie is sitting him up and propping pillows, etc.]

SUDDARDS: Does Joyce know?

JACKIE: Know what?

SUDDARDS: About the poker and drinking. She says I get brainless when I hang out with those guys. That's why I'm sleeping on the couch, I guess.

JACKIE: So, you got into a little trouble in the past, eh?

[Jackie continues fussing over Suddards, washes his hands and face with a cloth, rubs Suddards' feet and hands with lotion, puts his slippers on him, - all very tender, while instrumental version of "That Makes Me A Freak" plays underneath]

[Music stops]

JACKIE: How do you feel now, Mr. Suddards?

SUDDARDS: I feel like a new woman.

JACKIE: *[laughs]* Is that right? *[Shakes his head.]* Well, how about a shave madam?

[Jackie shaves Suddards, puts on cologne, combs his hair for him - again tenderly and silent, with same music behind]

SUDDARDS: I like you.

JACKIE: I like you too, sir.

SUDDARDS: You know you fooled me that first time.

JACKIE: How's that?

SUDDARDS: You were supposed to be a girl *[pause]* but you're a good boy. *[Looks directly into Jackie 's eyes.]* Yes, a mighty good boy.

JACKIE: Thank you sir. Now how about a new suit? *[Gets out some pajamas.]*

SUDDARDS: Are we going to church?

JACKIE: No, we're staying home today.

SUDDARDS: Well, don't tell mama. She says it's a sin to stay in bed.

JACKIE: It's our secret, sir.

[Jackie takes off Suddards' old pajama shirt, holds up clean pajama bottom. It is obviously way too large for the gaunt body in front of him.]

SUDDARDS: These are dad's...what's going on?

JACKIE: We'll just have to roll up the sleeves and cinch those pants a little.

SUDDARDS: I'm a big boy. "Jack, you're a big boy," mama always says, "a mighty big boy. Why you just grow out those pants like you was a weed." That's what she always says...

[Jackie finishes dressing Suddards]

JACKIE: Well, big boy, how about something to eat? *[puts bowl of soup in the microwave]*

SUDDARDS: Tacos *[He starts to say/sing a current taco restaurant ad]*

JACKIE: *[Laughs]* It's four o'clock in the morning so I don't think I'll be running out for Mexican right now. But I do have some soup. How about that?

[Microwave bell rings]

SUDDARDS: Company!

JACKIE: *[Getting soup out]* No, that's the oven.

SUDDARDS: Oh ya, bread. Must be Monday. She always bakes on Monday. Seven loaves for 7 days.

JACKIE: Sounds good, but the best I can do is this chicken broth. Here, try some. *[He holds a spoonful out to Suddards]*

SUDDARDS: Am I sick?

JACKIE: Yes.

SUDDARDS: Well, this will do the trick. I always get a sore throat after skating...Oh, oh, wet feet. Mentholatum too – that helps me breathe better. Yup, Vick's on a warm flannel cloth.

JACKIE: Well, this will warm you right up.

[Jackie keeps offering the soup, but Suddards doesn't really eat any. Eventually Suddards starts to nod off]

JACKIE: Are you tired Mr. Suddards?

SUDDARDS: Mentho...morphio...

JACKIE: Did I wear you out Mr. Suddards?

SUDDARDS: *[Looks around in confusion.]* What are we doing here?

JACKIE: Well, I like to call it the morphine chat.

[Jackie covers Suddards up.]

SUDDARDS: Good night sweetheart. (Falls asleep with face toward audience)

JACKIE: [smiles] Good night, sir.

SONG: Reprise of "That Makes Me a Freak"

[Darling in a spotlight on stage right, taking off her wig and looking at herself in mirror, Jackie is folding up Suddards' pajamas, Suddards is sitting in bed face forward propped up on pillows]

[Suddards and Darling sing]
And when I look at me now
I can't see what used to be
[Suddards] Where is that whole, firm flesh?
[Darling] and the curls blowing in the breeze?
[Suddards] Can I be a man?
[Darling] or a woman now?
[Suddards and Darling] or are we destined to be freaks?

[Sung by Jackie & Darling]
We never thought we could be so strong
to face death every day and not fall down.
We are freakish, set apart,
but our oddest trait
is a generous heart.
We never thought we could be so strong
to face death every day and not fall down.

[Sung by Jackie]
I'm a freak, I guess it's true
but just let me be

and I will take care of you.
I'm a freak, I guess it's true
but just let me be
and I will take care of you.

Scene 5 - Doctors and Gods

[Very soft lights come up on the examining room center stage. Dr. Deity and Dr. Franco are reviewing charts which are stacked up on the desk. Dr. Deity is seated at the desk, with desk lamp on, Dr. Franco is sitting in a chair with charts on his lap. All is silent as the scene opens.]

DR. DEITY: *[Takes off glasses, rubs his eyes, stretches and leans back.]* What time is it?

DR. FRANCO: *[Looks at his watch almost absentmindedly.]* It's twelve-thirty, sir.

DR. DIETY: Well, that's enough for today. We can't do anyone any good if we get too tired. When is the last time you slept?

DR. FRANCO: I caught a nap earlier. I'm OK. Didn't you want to review the Suddards' chart?

DR. DIETY: Oh, yes. But I think I know...

DR. FRANCO: Well, if anyone can change his prognosis...

DR. DEITY: It's not always possible.

DR. FRANCO: I know, but I have great faith in you and so does Mr. Suddards.

DR. DIETY: Why don't you get some rest. I'll look at the chart and if it's different from what we suspect I'll give you a nudge.

DR. FRANCO: Really? *[He moves the charts from his lap to the desk. He goes to the examining table and flops down on it]*   Ahhh... *[He falls immediately asleep]*

[Lights go down until it is just the desk lamp and one of the X-ray panels lit. Dr. Deity puts his glasses on and opens a chart and puts up an X-ray with the name Suddards on it. This is projected on the big screen. He stands to look closely at the X-ray. After a pause he shakes his head. He returns to the desk, gently closes the file and pats it]

DR. DIETY: Damn!

[Dr. Deity goes over to Dr. Franco, who is sound asleep. He gets a blanket out of a drawer and covers Dr. Franco up. Dr. Franco stirs]

DR. FRANCO: Doctor? What time?

DR. DEITY: There's nothing you can do now. We did what we could. Just get some rest.

SONG: Hush Now
Lyrics by Sara M. Slayton
Music by Hans Mayer

[Dr. Deity strokes Dr. Franco's hair as he sings the first verse]
I'm just a man
No matter what you think I am
I can't save every single one, single one
There is no cure
I must admit
I am alone
Hush now

[*Then he turns back to the X-ray panel* as he sings the second verse]

If I were God
I wouldn't need all of this would I?
I'd pick you up and stroke your hair
mend your wing,
set you off to fly.
I wish I was
what you think I am
I'm just a man
a child of God, like you.)

(Bridge)

[*During the instrumental bridge, soft lights come up on the Suddards Hospice Scene. Jackie is attending to Suddards whose breathing is very labored*]

[*Jackie and Dr. Deity sing both verses one more time. At the end, Jackie pulls the blanket over Suddards' face. Lights down on both sets.*]

JACKIE: Good night, sir.

Scene 6: Passing the Torch

[*Same radiation waiting room as in all other scenes, with these changes; a poster of two hands passing a torch is displayed (Olympic-like) and there is a new, healthy plant.*]

[*Dark stage except for aquarium light. Spot comes up on a female child sitting in Darling's chair. She just looks out at the audience. She is bald, but obviously female by her dress. Spot draws back and reveals mother seated next to her. The mother's face is obscured because she is busily filling out*

papers on a clipboard. There are three other patients in the
waiting room, but their faces are obscured too - one is behind
a magazine, one is napping with hat pulled down over face
and one is looking at the posters on the wall.]

[Darling enters. She has short, stubble hair and is wearing a
volunteer's jacket. She feeds the fish, makes coffee,
straightens magazines, etc. As she does she makes eye
contact with the girl. She smiles at her and waves to her. The
child is obviously curious, but shy. Darling gets out a watering
can and fills it at the sink. She goes over to water the plant.
The child silently approaches her.]

[Underneath this action an instrumental version of
"The Darling of the Waiting Room" plays softly]

[Music stops]

DARLING: Would you like to help? [She hands the watering
can to the child who waters the plant]

CHILD: Enough?

DARLING: Perfect. Now it will be fine.

[Darling walks over to the toy box and the child follows her.
She pulls out a few toys, holds them up and toward the
child...no reaction. Until she holds up the cowgirl doll. The
child smiles.]

DARLING: Would you like to play?

[Darling hands the doll to the child and kneels down in front
of her. The child strokes the doll's hair and dress.]

CHILD: I want to be a cowgirl when I grow up.

DARLING: Me too.

CHILD: We could be cowgirls together.

DARLING: Yes...together...*[pause]* That's a pretty dress.

CHILD: *[Looks at doll's dress, then her own.]* Pretty hair.
[Holds doll out to Darling.]

 DARLING: *[Touches doll]* It's pretty long. Not like mine, I like
to keep mine short. You too I see. *[Touches child's head.]*

CHILD: No, it's because I'm sick. But the doctor's gonna fix me.

DARLING: Ohh...*[she is at a loss for words]*

CHILD: *[Reaches into the toy box and pulls out a stuffed
dog]* Here. *[offers dog to Darling]* You can be my pet dog,
Rusty. When I get in trouble you can save me.

DARLING: OK, I'll try.

CHILD: You can do it I bet. *[Child resumes play]* Watch out! It's
a deep, dark hole. Oh no, I fell in. Come Rusty, here boy! Save
me...

*[Nurse enters and approaches the mother, bends over her,
murmurs, takes the papers]*

*[Mother rises and takes the child's hand and leads her toward
the radiation door.]*

CHILD: *[Hands the doll to Darling as she goes by her]*
I gotta go now, but we can play again.

[Child, Mother and Nurse exit]

DARLING: Yes we can, darling.

[Lights down. Darling stands alone in spot light and reprises the prologue, black & white photos from prologue projected]

DARLING: We were reluctant volunteers. But we had a captive audience, danced in over-sized heels, did magic tricks, sang songs, and accepted the applause. We were legends, my friends and I. What would we be? What adventures awaited us? What daring deeds? Our projections didn't include illness, only happy trails, and never an unhappy ending. We do the best we can, all of us. And we will play out our episodes, riding happy trails until we meet again.

[Music builds as the waiting room patients begin a reprise of "The Darling of the Waiting Room" song.]

[All cast comes on stage, using the 3 different sets, to sing and dance to the "Darling of the Waiting Room" – using the song as a curtain call. Any dual characters are revealed by projecting their 'other' faces on the X-ray panels as they take their bows.]
Finis

www.ingramcontent.com/pod-product-compliance
Lightning Source LLC
Chambersburg PA
CBHW070917290526
45795CB00001B/346